A gentle introduction to

Yoga

Revised Edition

Kareen Zebroff

foulsham

LONDON • NEW YORK • TORONTO • SYDNEY

Contents

What You Should Know

What exactly is yoga?

Most people these days have at least some idea as to what is hidden behind the word yoga. It is often linked with body control, rest, relaxation and balance. What is yoga, however, and how does it work?

The 'art' of yoga which originally came from India, is over 5,000 years old and was first written down about 2,500 years ago. It is, then, the oldest recorded exercise system for the conscious development of the human body and spirit. Basically, it is divided into two main areas: Hatha yoga with its asanas (body positions), and the yoga of meditation, of which there are different types.

In this book we are concerned with Hatha yoga, the only form of yoga that concerns itself with the body. Naturally, it is only a small part of the whole. But it is a very important one – Hatha yoga is the first step on the ladder leading to self-knowledge (Samadhi).

Yogi Sara Sangraha describes yoga in the following way: 'Soul and spirit become quiet and balanced through the mastery of the body and the feelings; the pathway leads to the becoming visible and the recognition of the true and highest being.' This 'true and highest being' can be described as the good in us, or as the image of God in us. Yoga shows us the way to the freedom of self, whatever the religion to which we belong. Yoga deepens it and gives to it more joy of living.

Only when one has mastery over the body can spirit and soul be free. A deepening within one's self can only be successful if there is no disturbance of bodily functions or if any pain distracts from meditation. In the same way that one can hardly notice the beauty of nature speeding by when one is sitting in a motor car and is disturbed by rattling noises or by a broken shock absorber, so it is just as difficult to concentrate on one's thoughts if the back or other muscles are in pain. Hatha yoga is directed towards organic health, not on the development of muscles (although this can be a side-effect). The secret of yoga is to stretch and contract the muscles and not, as in gymnastics, to put them under tension. The stretching exercises have been taken from cats. What do they do when they get up? They stretch themselves. Stretching means to relax and be at rest. In the case of yoga exercises all are done slowly and thoughtfully, so the slightest feeling of pain can bring everything to a standstill. These warning signs should be noted as the body seeks in this way to protect itself from strain and injury.

The meaning of yoga lies in personal advancement that cannot be measured against other people, but only against oneself – the self of the day before. This brings a feeling of success and certainty into your exercised, no matter what age you are, or how nimble and healthy. Only go as far in a position as *you* can

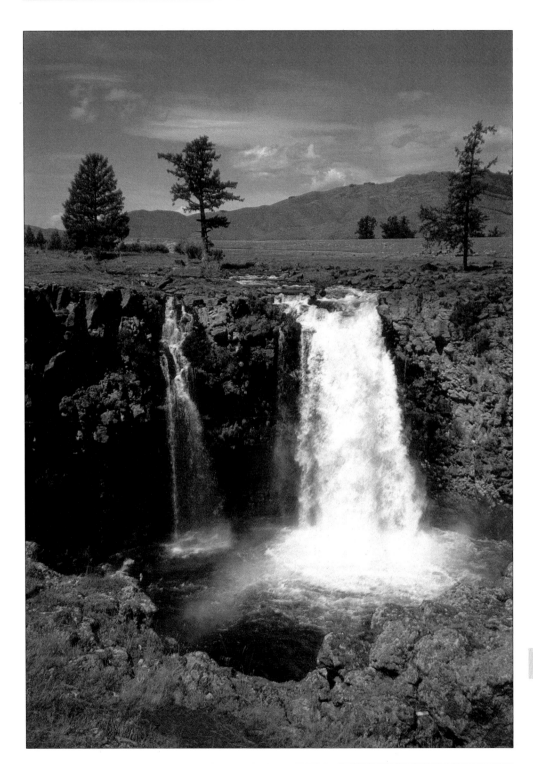

manage, and stay in this position until it becomes uncomfortable. By remaining in the position you exercise more intensively, and instead of doing an exercise 20 times you only need to do it two or three times. It relaxes and strengthens your muscles for the particular purpose you have chosen for yourself.

By regular half-hour exercises you can completely change your life! Yoga relaxes, makes one younger, brings more strength, stabilises and regulates the functioning of the body, gives energy and protects. It brings relief to digestion problems, haemorrhoids and all kinds of pain. There are special exercises for sciatica, slipped disc, bursitis and a lot more. Whether your legs hurt in the evening, whether you sleep badly or do not relax when sleeping, or whether you become easily annoyed or are not at peace with the world, yoga can help you!

For this book the 'pure' yoga teaching – in as far as has been thought necessary – has been changed a little. We live in the western world and right from our very first day we exposed to different influences than the Indians, for example. Our living conditions, our mentality and constitution differ so much from the way of life in the East that we have to accentuate the yoga exercises in a different way. The sense of yoga is not changed as we are still rewarded with rest and balance.

Why should we practise?

The aim of Hatha yoga is in the first place to keep the body healthy. The exercises are extended in their effect. They can keep you healthy throughout life and also increase your life expectation. The functions of your body and strength need not decline the older you get! If you keep up yoga on a regular basis, you will strengthen the whole organism. Depending upon the exercise, the bloodstream will be directed to particular organs, which will then be strengthened and regenerate themselves. Above all, a good blood circulation plays an important role in health and well-being.

According to the theory of evolution at one time we all moved about on 'all-fours'. In this position the heart lies under the spine, and almost the entire body finds itself horizontal. This makes it much easier for the blood to circulate to all parts of the body. Our position has altered in the process of development – we now walk upright. Following the law of gravity, the head is no longer properly circulated with blood. The stomach muscles lose their elasticity over the years, and the organs hang downwards and press against one another. The same is true of the muscles between the ribs connected to the skeleton – all are put under stress. The consequences are stomach troubles and back pain, and many other problems. The legs are also drawn into this suffering, they feel heavy and tend to develop varicose veins, no wonder then that the 'reverse' positions of yoga, such as the headstand and the Candle are good for the body. And an exercise such as pulling in the stomach each day is imperative to the maintenance of good health. As a result of these exercises, most of the organs in the stomach are brought back into their proper position – strong, massaged and strengthened. As a result of stimulating the circulation and the metabolism, problems such as indigestion get better and are eventually healed completely. Residues and poisons can more easily be flushed out, which builds up resistance to sickness and results in increased vitality.

Many yoga exercises have a particularly positive effect on the spine. This is especially important, as a straight and elastic spine is the basic requirement for concentration and relaxation. Extensive posture damage can be remedied through yoga. However, the spine is only part of the whole. No part of the body is independent of the other. All organs stand in a permanent interrelation; every bodily process releases another. In the case of mental or physical strain, for example, muscles will contract so that they do not function properly. This contraction of the muscles paralyses tendons and ligaments – the joints become stiff. The result: you feel unwell, have no energy, are irritated, tense and depressed. This disastrous circle can be broken with yoga. For many sicknesses and complaints there are special exercises that will bring relief in a very short time, and at the same time there are no unpleasant side-effects! Before turning to medicines, you should first try the appropriate yoga exercises. This naturally applies only to minor health complaints. In the case of more serious complaints the advice of a doctor should be sought. If you breathe properly during the exercises and really relax, you will soon discover that yoga not only helps you to obtain a healthy body but also gives you energy and provides harmony and joy of living.

At one time I was myself 25 pounds overweight and completely discouraged. I lived in an area in the extreme north of Canada together with my children, all three under five years old, and I felt perpetually tired and under the weather. The children were sickly and contacts in the area were unsatisfying. I grew increasingly sorry for myself. My problems were not even hidden from my mother. In a letter she told me how much good yoga had done her as she entered the menopause, and she encouraged me to take it up and discover it for myself.

I did just that, and it completely changed my life. As a result of the yoga exercises and a sensible diet – plenty of protein, few carbohydrates – I lost my surplus weight in three months. My energy increased daily, and I saw the world through different eyes. My children also benefited (once more they had a patient, loving mother). I took over my household with both hands, with energy and concentration. My posture and appearance improved, I felt prettier, and I was too. My body became more elastic and recovered its shape. I lost centimetres everywhere, even on the inside of the thighs which were always a cause of concern to me. People told me I looked years younger. But far better than this was the feeling of freshness, of being alive – a feeling of being wide-awake to develop my personality and say 'yes' to life completely. Now a day without my yoga exercises is for me incomplete.

Nutrition

A wholefood diet assumes that all food is consumed as near as possible to its natural state. Processed white flour should be taken out of the diet altogether and substituted by wholemeal flour. As a sweetener, instead of white refined sugar use honey. A balanced diet, consisting of dairy produce, fish, fruit, vegetables and cereal products, already contains a sufficient quantity of carbohydrates. A supplement of carbohydrates (e.g. in the form of sugar) is therefore, totally unnecessary. Vegetables should only be steamed or stewed for as long as it takes for them not to lose their crispiness. Even better, eat them raw. Natural rice still in its husk is always preferable to polished white rice as the husk contains many valuable vitamins and minerals. Noodles and all cakes and pastries should be made from wholemeal flour. Also nuts, dried fruit and yoghurt should be included in the diet plan. In the case of fruit vegetables and cereals, care should be taken that they have been grown organically.

As a general rule all foods that have been heavily processed should be avoided, such as refined foods (e.g. sugar or instant foods), foods containing artificial additives, and those having undergone chemical changes (e.g. hardened fats).

For the yogi, the body is the temple of the soul and therefore there is the responsibility of remaining healthy. This is because, according to his standpoint, the body has the purpose of housing the spirit and everything must be avoided that lies heavy upon the soul and makes it lethargic. A yogi will eat a small snack frequently during the day, but only when he is hungry. He chews thoroughly and eats slowly. He knows that digestion starts in the mouth, where the enzymes in the saliva set in motion the first of the many digestive processes. These small meals can consist of shoots and sprouts, a little yoghurt, a little piece of cheese, a banana or dried fruit with nuts. A yogi will never eat a very rich meal – he is moderate in all things. He always makes sure that his diet contains sufficient protein. This is why he will often eat seeds, soya beans, wheat sprouts, nuts and dairy products.

A balanced diet with lots of fresh fruit and vegetables deepens and supports the positive effects of the yoga exercises upon body and soul. If, in addition, you want to reduce weight, we recommend a low-calorie diet with sufficient added vitamins and minerals. They play an important role in the metabolic process and take care of the natural dehydration of the cells.

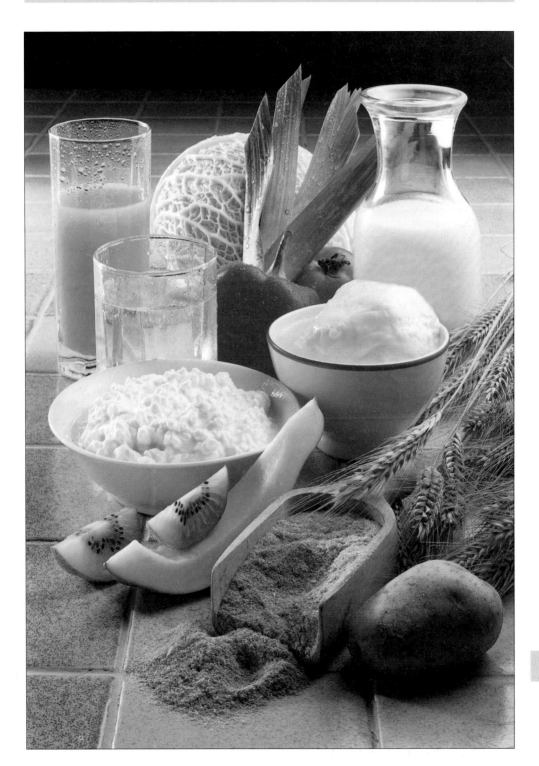

How the yoga exercises should be done

Everyone expects something different from yoga. One person may be mostly concerned about the figure, which needs improvement here and there. Another may be looking for more energy, and wants to lose a few pounds. Older people, who feel that they are getting a little stiff, will be looking for something to ease their aches and pains. They know that something must be done in order to regain that feeling of vitality, and to once more experience how good food can taste, and how restful sleep can be. Taking all these requirements together, we have the collective expression *health*, but also that of *work*. The beautiful thing about yoga is that the effort required does not seem like effort. The results are truly remarkable, but they do not tire one out. Even after the most energetic yoga exercises, the muscles do not become stiff if the rules are carefully followed. In order to obtain the maximum effect with the minimum exertion in pursuing yoga, it is best to follow these basic rules.

Time

The best time for yoga is either immediately after getting up or just before going to bed – whatever best fits in with your daily routine! In the morning the body is stiff, but the exercises will give you energy and a good start to the day. In the evening the exercises are easier, they freshen you up, relax you and ensure that you sleep well. Whichever time you choose, make sure your stomach, bladder and bowels are relatively empty before you begin.

Place

The best place is an airy spot where you can be undisturbed. Then the more you concentrate on the exercises the more successful they will be. The ground should not be too soft; a carpet or a blanket folded several times on the floor is sufficient.

Hygiene

If you have gout or rheumatism, you should take a bath. Do the same when you are tense. Empty the bladder and the bowels before beginning the exercises. If you regularly do yoga, you will no longer suffer from constipation. The positions that are upside down encourage this emptying, so it is a good idea to do these kind of exercises right at the beginning.

Food

You should not do any of the exercises for at least two hours after eating heavily and about one hour after a light snack.

Cautions

Provided you follow the instructions carefully, the yoga exercises in this book are safe for most people. However, certain exercises are best avoided during the first days of menstruation and the last five months of pregnancy, and in conditions such as serious heart trouble. *Whenever necessary, a cautionary note is given after the instructions for the exercise.*

For the ladies

You can do yoga even when you have your period, as long as you do not overdo things and the strength of the bleeding does not change suddenly. You should not do exercise upside down, such as the Candle. For the first three months of pregnancy you can do yoga without any worries, but you should speak to your doctor about it. There are special exercises that make giving birth easier. These strengthen the back muscles and make them more elastic. There are also exercises that strengthen the base of the hips and enable you to breathe deeply.

High blood pressure, dizzy spells and detached retina

Anyone suffering from any of these things must first consult a doctor. At the beginning you should not do any exercises upside down such as the Candle. As the inverted posture progresses, the veins extend and dizziness or headache may be experienced. In standing forward bends, the head should not be taken lower than the heart, so bend only halfway and do not hold the posture. As a result of the upside-down position, the veins extend. This will lead to a sudden and strong rush of blood to the head, which can lead to headaches and dizziness.

Yoga asanas (positions)

There is no doubt that yoga can work miracles. In the end it will be through you yourself that the miracles occur. Without your discipline, without your belief in what you are doing, and without the patience, there an be no results. One can practise yoga correctly or incorrectly; it is often because of a tiny deviation that the exercise does not work. Read the instructions thoroughly and to the end. Many people listen with only half an ear and look only at the tail end of the instructions. The exercises will appear just the same. Whatever your age, yoga can help you to fulfil the secret dreams about your body. Whether what you desire is more energy, health, beauty or better posture, you will receive it, if you practise yoga regularly and sensibly.

How much to do of the yoga asanas

1. Practise yoga regularly, even if on some days you can only do a few exercises owning to pressure of time. Choose those which you know exactly will do *you* some good. If you are, for example, under stress, then do the chest expander. If your stomach troubles you, then do the pump. Practise yoga with the same regularity as eating and sleeping! You will be rewarded with health and a new outlook on life.

2. Take your time. Take up the position only very slowly. Take 10 to 15 seconds, until you reach the final position. This is much better for your body and makes the exercise much more effective. Besides this, you will then not have to repeat the exercises so often.

3. Many postures can be repeated two or three times but should then be held until you become uncomfortable. The tension on the muscles must increase so that they keep their shape. As a beginner, you should remain in the position for about five seconds; this can be increased weekly by a further five seconds. Remaining in the position has the same effect as if it were continually repeated. For this reason it is sufficient to do the exercised just three instead of 20 times.

4. End the position just as slowly as you started it. If you don't, the exercise will lose at least a third of its value and there is also the danger of injuring yourself. So, always perform the exercise nice and slowly.

5. Do not force anything. Do not make any jerky movements just in order to reach further or deeper. Go just as far as you can and persevere there. Pain is the alarm signal of the body. Do not be deaf to it. Always listen to it, otherwise you will injure yourself. If you move yourself too quickly, if the movements are too quick, then you will run into danger of missing the alarm signals.

6. Never compare yourself with others! With yoga the important thing is your own personal success. If you do your yoga exercises regularly, then you will be a little better than the day before. When you reach the full extent of what is possible for you, then you will achieve the same effect as a deeper bend performed by someone else somewhat more supple. In yoga only your own success if of importance. After some time you will master positions you never thought were possible.

7. Concentrate fully on the exercise that you are doing at the time, then it will work. Concentration is particularly important in the case of the balancing exercises. Quick movements of the head, speaking, or slight embarrassed laughter when one loses balance reduces the effectiveness. Continue quietly on from where you broke off, and do not let yourself be overwhelmed by a sense of discouragement or failure. Follow the exercise carefully through as this strengthens the concentration, and this again will help you to do the exercise better. In the case of the Lion, pretend to be a wild lion, and at another time a little kitten that has just woken from its afternoon nap. Then the exercises will be a lot more fun!

8. Have a rest between exercises. The attraction of yoga lies in its gentleness. You do not need to suffer from tiredness or muscle strain. Stop from time to time, so that your muscles have the chance to relax again. Give your body the chance to adjust to anything new.

9. Breathe as normally as possible when remaining in the position. Many people believe that they must hold their breath while they desperately hold a cramped position. This is completely wrong. Yoga makes you relaxed during the exercises. Go as far in any exercise as is possible without strain or pain, then relax and breathe as normally as possible. Every time you breathe out you can begin the exercise again. Breathing plays an important part in the success of an exercise. Please observe the following basic rules:
- Every time you raise your arm, breathe in.
- Every time you commence an exercise, breathe out.
- Every time you exert effort, breathe out strongly!

This also naturally means that first of all you breathe in, and then the most energetic part is done while breathing out. This applies, for example, to the pelvis stretch (stage 5), Bow (stage 4), Fish (stage 2), Grasshopper (stage 2), Camel (stage 4), Candle (stage 2), knee and ankle stretching (stage 4), Pump (stage 3). One exception is the Cobra. Breathe *in* when beginning the exercise, and breathe *out* when coming out of the position. First, become fully acquainted with the course of an exercise before you consider the breathing techniques.

Breath control

Hatha yoga consists of three components: the exercises, the cleansing of the body, and breath control. Out of these three the yogis give pre-eminence to control of breathing, as air is the most important food for body, soul and spirit. In the language of the yogis, Sanskrit, breath control is called *Pranayama*. *Prana* means breath of living energy and *ayama* means to hold or control. The yogis believe that the invisible cosmic power all around us provides us with an invisible and mysterious source of life. Without prana we would all be dead; the more we have of it, the more vitality and energy there will be in us. A a result of breath control we can increase of life energy. We become awake and conscious of the self, and we learn self-control.
If you were to conduct a scientific experiment on yourself, you would discover that you can live for over a month without solid food, for a week without liquids and sleep, but only for a few minutes without oxygen. Even if you make a conscious decision not to breathe (small children do this sometimes in order to get their way), you would soon lose consciousness

and exactly at that point begin to breathe again. It is amazing how strong our unconscious control of breathing is, and without it we would not be able to express our feelings in terms of laughter, tears, shrieks and sighs. The way we breathe can have a lot of influence on the world of our feelings, which is evident from a very simple observation. If we are excited or nervous, we breathe much faster than when we are resting. On the other hand, we can quieten ourselves down by taking a few deep breaths. Breathing properly quietens the soul, refreshes the spirit and lengthens the life, because the heart does not have to beat so often. It is good for the digestion, refreshes the complexion, purifies the blood and brings new energy. In order to understand all this it is necessary to understand how the process of breathing works. Oxygen fulfils two important functions in our bodies. Each one of the millions of cells must breathe, in order with the help of oxygen to renew themselves and to expel the used-up waste products (carbon dioxide). Oxygen is also needed to turn food into energy. On the other hand, the more you are full of energy the more oxygen you will require. Normally, on breathing in, the body will take in about a quarter of a litre of oxygen, which it takes at a rate of 5 litres per minute. The lungs can contain 5–6 litres of air. But you will usually, even at this very minute, only fill your lungs to about a fifth of their capacity. We must also learn how to breathe properly. From a technical point of view it happens as follows.

Our lungs expand and contract like a bladder, up to 20 times a minute. The muscle responsible for expansion and contraction is called the diaphragm. It has the shape of a dome. When it contracts, the lungs fill up and in doing this uses the muscles between the ribs. This stretches the chest, as a result of which the air can reach the extremities of the lungs. In order for the diaphragm to contract, it is necessary for the stomach to extend outwards. Unfortunately, most people do the opposite when breathing in. They pull in the stomach, and this is completely wrong. Correct breathing can be learned and the following advice should be heeded in all the breathing exercises:

1. Always breathe through the nose, which has the function of a filter. The air is warmed as it passes through the nose, dampened and freed of impurities. A well-known yogi once said: 'The mouth is for eating and kissing, the nose for breathing.'

2. Always sit completely upright so that the chest is not squeezed up. For asthmatics I recommend the Fish position, in which the head is thrown right back in order to ease breathing.

3. Do your breathing exercises either in a warm, well-ventilated room, or out of doors in warm, pollution-free air.

4. Ten minutes' slow, even breathing a day will be most valuable, creating energy, balance of character and cheerfulness.

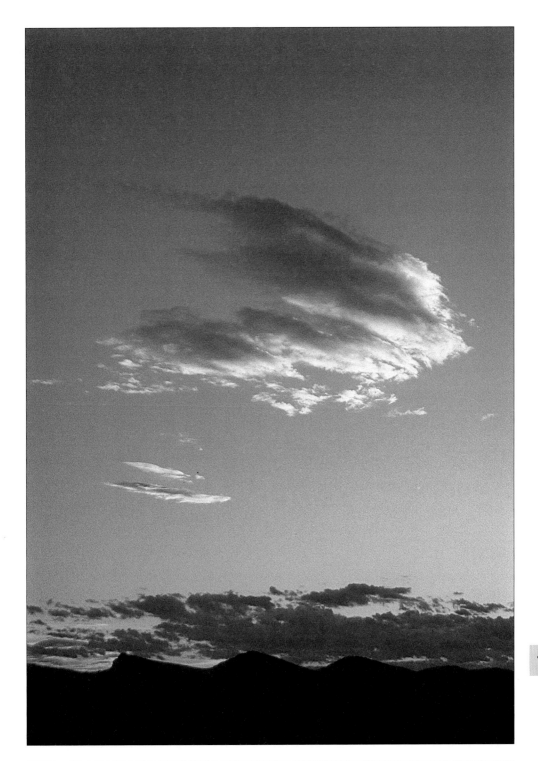

5. To hold your breath, cut it off by bending your head forwards and pressing the chin down onto the collarbone. After about five seconds, lift your head and breathe out. do not hold your breath if you suffer from high or low blood pressure or a heart condition.

6. Try to breathe gently and quickly in the beginning. Later you will have to make specific sounds with your breathing.

7. Movements of the body and breathing should follow the same rhythm, gently and slowly. This is the most effective way.

8. When breathing in, concentrate on relaxing the navel area and gently expanding the rib cage up to the armpits.

9. When breathing out, pull in the abdomen gently in order to push out as much air as possible.

The Yoga Asanas

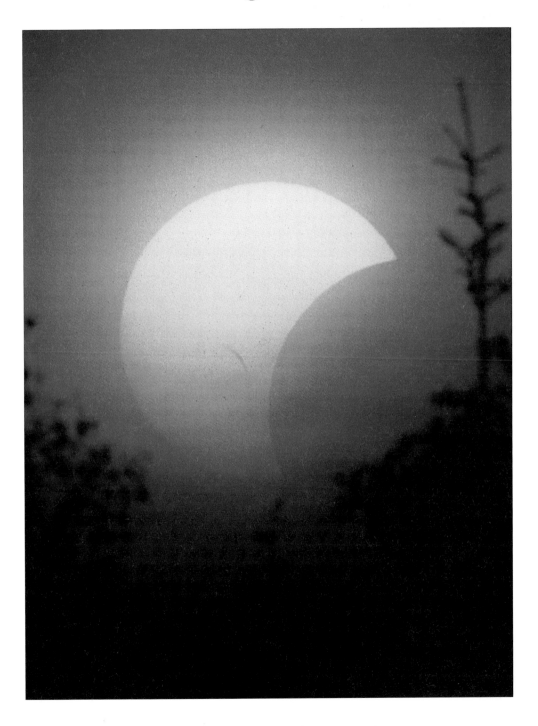

Lifting the arms

I. What the exercise is good for

Lifting the arms
- makes the flabby under-arm firm
- strengthens and firms the chest muscles
- relieves tense shoulders

II. How to do it

1. Sit comfortably in the 'tailor' position.
2. Lift your arms up to shoulder height, with the palms of the hands upwards, the fingers in the direction of the neck and the elbows facing outwards. Your arms make a straight line, parallel with the chest (Fig. 1).
3. Lift your hands slowly though at the same time resisting the movement, until your hands are as far up as they will go (Fig. 2).
4. Stretch out your arms, and lower your hands once more with the same contrary pressure. Breathe during the exercise as normally as possible.
5. Repeat the exercise three to five times.

III. This is the right way

Imagine for a moment that you must lift a heavy weight up over your head. This will help you to carry out the exercise properly. And you must lower it just as slowly. Imagine that the weight will otherwise crush you. Press against it firmly, so that the tendons of the arms and fingers appear. Rest if you can between the exercises and breathe normally. If you have just lost weight or are intending to do so, bear in mind that the evidence of this will show itself, especially under the arms.

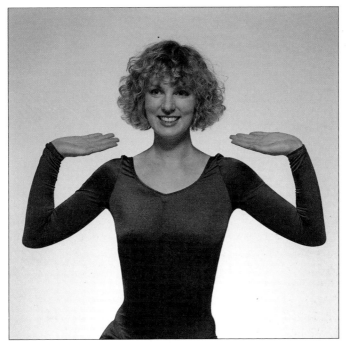

Fig. 1

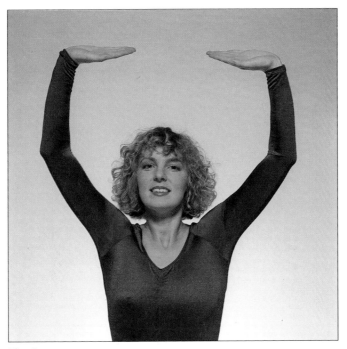

Fig. 2

Arm and leg stretching (Natarajasana)

I. What the exercise is good for

Arm and leg stretching
- stretches and tightens the whole front of the body
- encourages and protects body posture as it develops balance
- helps to relax the back and the thighs
- is a particularly pleasant massage for the vertebrae of the back because of the gentle stretching backwards
- stretches the chest

II. How to do it

1. Stand upright, heels together, with the toes pointed slightly outwards.
2. Lift the right arm slowly, until the hand is above your head. The elbow is straight.
3. Bend your left leg, and bring it to near your bottom. Put all your body weight onto the right foot.
4. Take hold of the left foot with the left hand (Fig. 3).
5. Bend yourself backwards from the waist, pulling on your foot at the same time and moving your right arm as far as you can backwards without falling over.
6. Remain in this position for 5 seconds, and lengthen the time by 5 seconds each week.
7. Do this exercise now with the other leg, and repeat it three times on each side.

III. This is the right way

If you experience difficulty in keeping your balance, then practise as easier ·balancing position like the Tree (see page 30).
Concentrate intensely during this exercise (this will help you keep your balance). As with all yoga exercises, you should move only slowly. Do not close you eyes while doing this exercise.

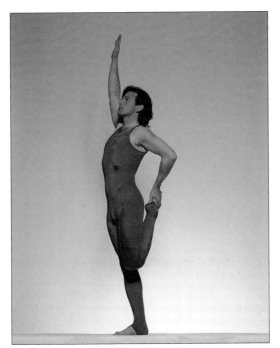

Fig. 3

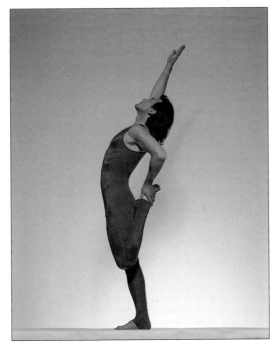

Fig. 4

Head-and-trunk raising

I. What the exercise is good for

Head-and-trunk raising
- strengthens the back, safely
- is one of the best exercises for strengthening and tightening the stomach muscles
- firms and tightens the bottom

II. How to do it

1. Lie down on your back. Your knees will be bent just enough for your feet to be flat on the floor.
2. Place your hands on your thighs and pull in your lower abdominal muscles (Fig. 5).
3. Slowly lift your head and trunk until it is roughly at an angle of 30 degrees. Your hands should in the meantime slide along the upper thighs towards the knees. Depending on the length of your arms, you should just about be able to touch your kneecaps (Fig. 6).
4. Remain in this position for 5–30 seconds.
5. Slowly take your head and trunk back down to the floor. Relax.
6. Repeat this exercise three or four times.

III. This is the right way

Do not lift the body up more than 30 degrees. If the exercise is too easy, this means that the muscles in the lower part of the body are not taut and so you have most certainly done the exercise incorrectly.
While doing this exercise breathe as normally as possible.
Sitting up is an excellent exercise for tightening the stomach and getting it back into shape, even a fat stomach. Unfortunately, all exercises for the stomach are tiring; if you repeat it regularly you will achieve quick and good results.

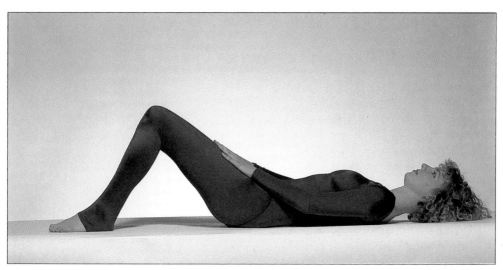

Fig. 5

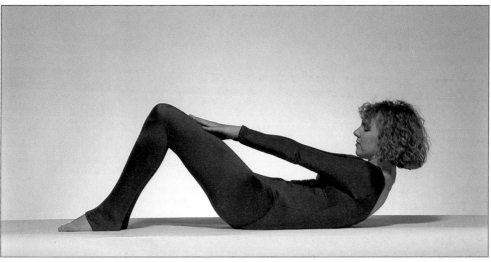

Fig. 6

Rolling the eyes

I. What the exercise is good for

Rolling the eyes
- helps when the eyes are tense and over-tired
- strengthens the eye muscles
- relieves headaches
- makes the eyes clear and shining
- has a generally relaxing effect

II. How to do it

1. Sit comfortably in the 'tailor' position, and look straight ahead.
2. Look as far as possible to the right without moving the head. Remain in this position for 5 seconds (Fig. 7).
3. Look as far as possible to the left without moving the head, again for 5 seconds (Fig. 8).
4. Look upwards under your eyebrows for 5 seconds (Fig. 9).
5. Look downwards along your nose. Remain like this again for 5 seconds (Fig 10).
6. Place a large clock in front of you so that the figure 12 is directly under your eyebrows and the 6 is directly on the floor in front of you.
7. Turn your eyes to follow the figures round, one figure per second, so that your eyes move with little jerks just like a second hand.
8. Repeat this in the opposite direction.
9. Cover your eyes with the palm of the hands for 30 seconds to rest them (Fig. 11).

III. This is the right way

Do this exercise when you are tired, or if you have been using your eyes a lot. Do not just rub them as you have probably done previously. Rest your eyes between the different exercises by shutting them.
The eyes are the most important of our sensory organs. Most of us neglect them and take their functioning without difficulties for granted. Eye tension and the resulting headaches can be avoided through these exercises.

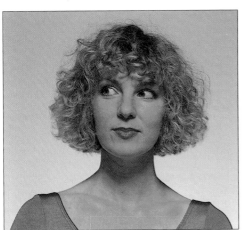
Fig. 7

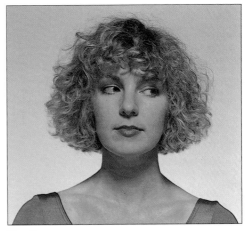
Fig. 8

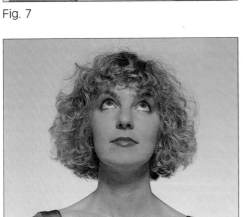
Fig. 9

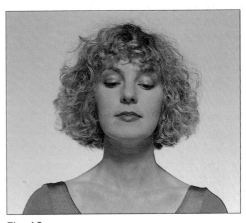
Fig. 10

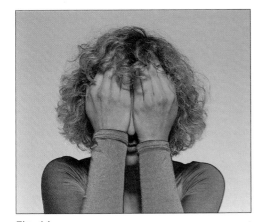
Fig. 11

Variations

1. a) Look out of the window into the distance. Try to look miles away to the horizon. Remain like this.
   b) Slowly bring your gaze back, and look cross-eyed towards your nose.

2. Give free rein to your imagination. For example, describe a half-circle with your eyes and all kinds of other shapes too – anything that comes to mind.

Pulling in the stomach (Uddiyana Bandha)

I. What the exercise is good for

Pulling in the stomach
- strengthens and firms the stomach muscles
- produces a slim waistline
- helps a regular digestion and prevents constipation through a stimulation of intestinal peristalsis
- Strengthens and massages the organs and glands of the abdomen
- encourages the blood circulation in the whole abdomen and works positively on the digestion

II. How to do it

1. Stand up straight with the feet about 1 foot (30 cm) apart.
2. Bend forwards and place the hands exactly above the knees. Rest your whole weight here.
3. Breathe in deeply and out deeply. Do not breathe again throughout the whole exercise. It is very important to empty the lungs as much as possible throughout this exercise.
4. Relax the stomach and pull it inwards and upwards as though the navel were to touch the spine. This will produce a deep hollow (Fig. 12).
5. Hold this pulling in of the stomach for a few seconds and then suddenly release it again (Fig. 13).
6. Quickly pull the stomach inwards and upwards again. The upwards pull should be strong enough to tighten the neck muscles.
7. After a second, let the stomach suddenly go again.
8. Repeat the pulling in and release of the stomach three to five times while holding the outward breath.
9. Relax and breathe in smoothly. If after having done the exercise you have to breathe out, then you have not done it properly.
10. Do this exercise three times, one after another. If you have digestion problems or the stomach muscles have been stretched, then the whole exercise should be done three times each day.

III. This is the right way

You must ensure that your lungs are empty before pulling in the stomach. This takes a little practice because of the tendency always to breathe in when pulling in the stomach. The whole cycle of three to five pull-ins must be done while holding the breath once. Make sure that your stomach is quite relaxed so that the hollow is produced successfully. Increase the cycle to 10 times within one holding of the breath, but do this only a step at a time (one more each week).
Do not become discouraged if your stomach is too fat and no hollow is to be detected. It takes a little while before the desired appearance can be achieved, but you will eventually do it.

Caution. Only practise this exercise on an empty stomach. Avoid it during menstruation, in pregnancy, and if you have high blood pressure, a stomach ulcer or a hernia.

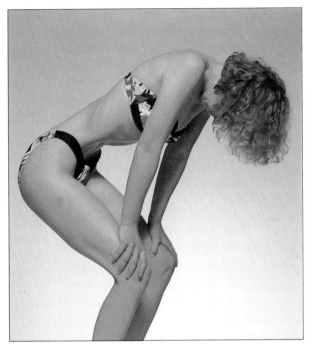

Fig. 12

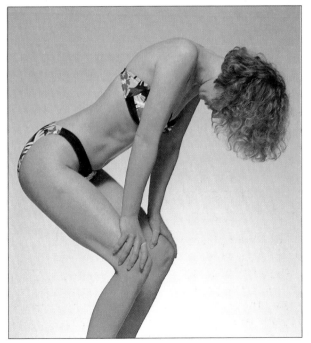

Fig. 13

The Tree (Vrksasana)

I. What the exercise is good for

The Tree
- encourages blood circulation to the lower extremities of the body
- produces a more graceful posture through a better balance
- improves the posture generally as the body must be held in an absolutely straight position in order not to fall over
- strengthens the stomach muscles

II. How to do it

1. Stand with the feet close together. The arms should be outstretched sideways.
2. Bend the right knee inwards, and bring the sole of your foot up to your left thigh.
3. Take the heel up as far as it will go, and stay there. The knee is pointing sideways (Fig. 14).
4. Place your palms on top of each other, and lift your hands outstretched above the head (Fig. 15).
5. Balance as long as you can, and breathe deeply.
6. Lower the heels and the hands quite slowly, and relax.
7. Repeat the exercise with the left foot.
8. Repeat the exercise twice on each side.

III. This is the right way

Support your foot more towards the front of the upper thigh, then it will not slip. Practise balancing first by holding the arms out sideways.
Do not come out of the position too quickly.
In the same way, the muscles also need practice in balancing in order to function – only balancing in this case will be successful more quickly. Do this balancing practice as often as you can, e.g. when answering the telephone.

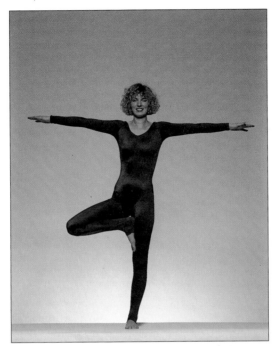

Fig. 14

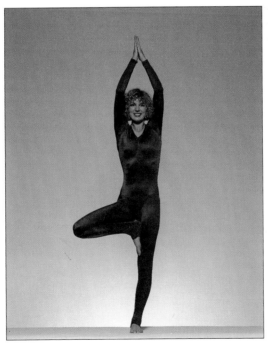

Fig. 15

Pelvis stretching
(Supta Virasana)

I. What the exercise is good for

Pelvis stretching
- relieves tension
- stretches and firms the legs, thighs and stomach
- strengthens back and legs
- stimulates the functioning of the glands and abdominal organs
- develops the chest muscles
- improves posture
- minimises fat build-up on the back of the legs and firms them

II. How to do it

1. Kneel down and sit on the heels with the feet together (Fig. 16).
2. Place your right hand behind you on the floor. The fingers point backwards and as a result the elbows are straight. In the same way place the left hand on the other side. Both hands rest in a straight line from the shoulders to the floor. Let your head hang backwards (fig. 17).
3. Press your pelvis now forwards and upwards as far as you can. Remain in this position 5–30 seconds (Fig. 18).
4. Lower the pelvis slowly in the position of a 'rolled-up leaf' (see page 116). The head rests on the floor, the chest against the knees, the bottom rests on the heels and the arms lie on the body.
5. Repeat the exercise, trying to place the hands further back. Then return to the position of the 'rolled-up leaf'.

6. Do this exercise three times altogether.

III. This is the right way

Do not forget to press your pelvis upwards, and your bottom should not be resting on your heels. Your whole body should be arched. Every time you do this exercise you should bend your body forwards in order to balance the extreme bending backwards. Given time you will be able to support yourself on your elbows and shoulders (Fig. 19). This asana is especially good to relieve female problems and pains.

Caution. Avoid this exercise during menstruation or in pregnancy. Omit it also if you have a heart condition, high blood pressure, arthritis of the neck joints or whiplash injury.

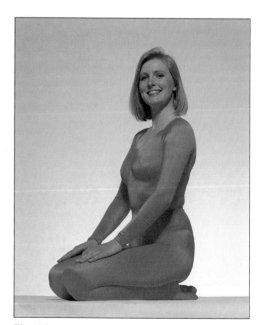

Fig. 16

32

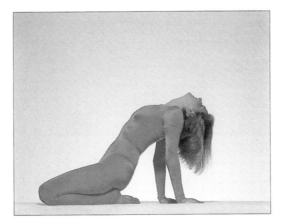

Fig. 17

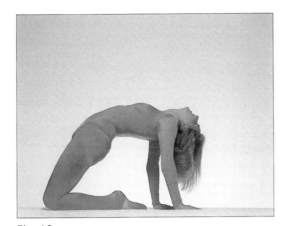

Fig. 18

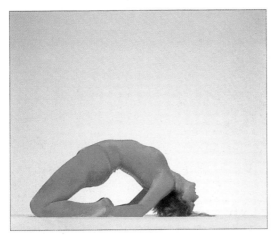

Fig. 19

Crossing over the legs (Crocodile) (Jatara Parivartanasana)

I. What the exercise is good for

The Crocodile
- removes fat layers
- massages the liver, pancreas and spleen and encourages them to function
- encourages digestion and relieves gastritis (stomach membrane infection)
- firms and shapes abdominal organs
- removes congestion in the lower part of the back and thighs

II. How to do it

1. Lie down on your back, arms stretched out to the side.
2. Lift your right leg slowly, keeping it straight until it is pointing vertically upwards (Fig. 20).
3. Move the leg to the left, away from the body, and try to reach the floor with the foot.
4. Be careful to keep both shoulders firmly on the floor, even if you have to resort to gripping the leg of a chair with the left hand.
5. As soon as you have brought the leg as far as you can in the direction of the floor, turn your head to the right (Fig. 21).
6. Remain in this position for 5–20 seconds.
7. Lift your leg up high again slowly, and then bring it back to the starting position again. (If necessary, bend the leg as you do this.)
8. Do the same thing with the other leg.
9. Repeat the exercise with both legs parallel (Fig. 22).

Variation: Bend your legs and then lower them to the side.

III. This is the right way

Do not roll onto your side when bringing down your leg. Remain with your shoulders firmly on the ground in order to effect a sideways movement of the spine.
Always turn your head in the opposite direction to the leg.

Caution. Do not do this exercise during menstruation or in pregnancy.

34

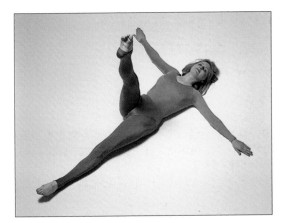

Fig. 20

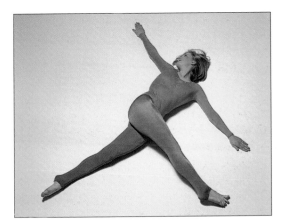

Fig. 21

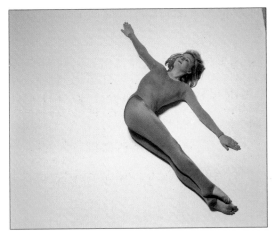

Fig. 22

Mountain (Parvatasana)

I. What the exercise is good for

The Mountain
- relaxes the nervous system
- encourages the digestion and prevents constipation
- builds and firms the stomach muscles and abdomen
- strengthens the spine
- strengthens the lungs and enriches the blood with oxygen
- relieves tension

II. How to do it

1. Sit down comfortably with a completely straight back in the 'tailor' position.
2. Place the palms of the hands together in front of your chest as though praying (Fig. 23).
3. Press the palms in front of your chest together, at the same time stretching the arms above the head (Fig. 24).
4. In order to stretch a little further, imagine that you want to touch the sky with your fingertips (Fig. 25).
5. Stay in this position from 5 to 30 seconds. Breathe normally.
6. Lower your arms quite slowly.
7. Relax.
8. This exercise can also be done as a breathing exercise.

III. This is the right way

Keep your back quite straight while doing this exercise so that it does the back some good.
Do not hold your breath.
In this exercise appearance are deceptive. Even those who mock are forced to admit that it is more difficult than it appears. If the stretching is done properly, this has a very relaxing effect.

Caution. Omit this posture if you have venous clots in your legs.

36

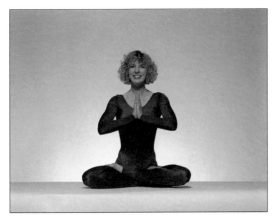

Fig. 23

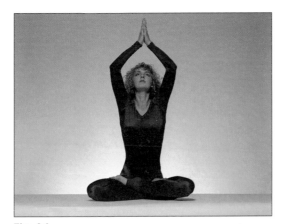

Fig. 24

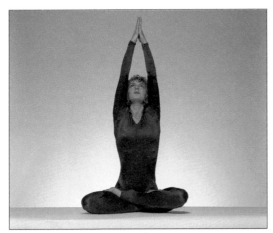

Fig. 25

Flower

I. What the exercise is good for

The Flower
- helps painful joints and loosens stiff fingers
- prevents weakness in the joints
- gives the hands a youthful appearance
- assists a good blood circulation
- makes and keeps the fingers supple for piano playing, typing and all kinds of hand work

II. How to do it

1. Sit comfortably in the 'tailor' position.
2. Make the hand into a fist, and press quite hard (Fig. 26).
3. Imagine that your hand is a flower that opens itself in the morning sun and try with a strong contrary pressure to open your hands slowly (Fig. 27).
4. Bend your fingers as far as possible backwards (Fig. 28).
5. Close your hands with the same contrary pressure with which you opened them. The pressure must be strong enough to make the tendons on the back of the hand stand out.
6. Relax the fingers by moving them quickly or shaking them.
7. Next spread out the fingers, and press each finger one at a time against the palm of the hand. Remain like this for 2 seconds each time.
8. Repeat the whole exercise twice.

III. This is the right way

Do the exercise in warm water or oil – the effect is the same, but it will not hurt. For anyone with inflamed joints it is very important that these joints do not become stiff. These exercises also contribute to beauty – they keep the hands looking young. Often it is the hands that give away age.

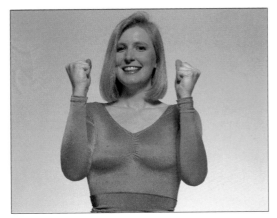

Fig. 26

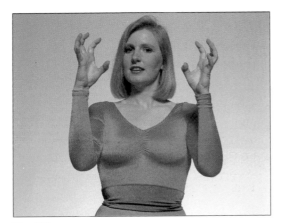

Fig. 27

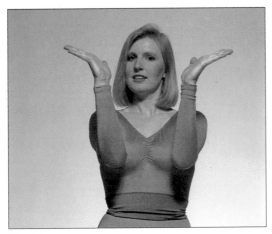

Fig. 28

Bow (Dhanurasana)

This is a more advanced exercise so should be avoided by complete beginners.

I. What the exercise is good for

The Bow
- ▶ relieves the pain of a slipped disc
- ▶ builds and firms muscles in the stomach, arms, legs and in the back
- ▶ develops and firms the chest and chest muscles
- ▶ strengthens the spine and makes it supple
- ▶ reduces build-up of fat round the thighs and bottom
- ▶ aids digestion
- ▶ improves posture

II. How to do it

1. Lie on your stomach on the floor, with arms and legs alongside the body.
2. Bend the knees and bring them as near as possible to your bottom.
3. Grasp your ankles, first the one, then the other (Fig. 29).
4. Lift your knees from the floor by pulling the ankles away from the hands. Your hands must still hold tightly onto the ankles, but as a result of the pulling away it will be easier for you to lift your knees from the floor than by pulling down.
5. Lift up your head at the same time (Fig. 30).
6. Remain for 5 to 10 seconds in this position at the beginning, and increase it at a rate of 5 seconds per week up to 30 seconds. Breathe as normally as possible all through.
7. Reach the final position only very slowly, relax and then rest a short while.
8. Repeat the exercise twice.

III. This is the right way

Only come out of the position very slowly. Pull the ankles 'high and away', not downwards, in order to get obstinate knees off the ground. Do not bounce quickly back otherwise a third of the effect will be lost. This exercise demands a lot from you, but returns a good deal in usefulness. This is a daily 'must' in your programme.

Caution. This exercise is not suitable for absolute beginners. Also avoid practising the Bow if you have a heart condition, a hernia or if you are pregnant.

40

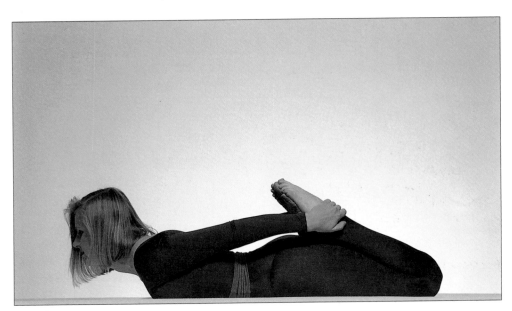

Fig. 29

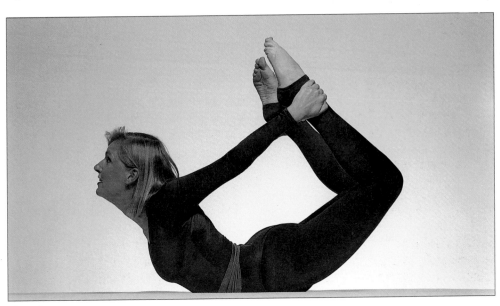

Fig. 30

41

Windmill

I. What the exercise is good for

The Windmill
▷ tightens and removes flab from thighs
▷ makes a slimmer waistline
▷ encourages good circulation in the arms
▷ stretches the body on both sides
▷ relaxes

II. How to do it

1. Stand with feet slightly apart and parallel. Do not turn the toes out. Fold the hands hanging down in front of the body.

2. Slowly lift the folded hands above the head and move the pelvis forward and down. Lift your breast bone and stretch backwards as far as you can. Do not lean back from the waist – stretch your spine. Stay in this position for a few seconds (Fig. 31).

3. With your body, describe a circle from the waist by bending first to the left and forwards and then to the right. Remain in each bend for a few seconds (Figs. 32 and 33). Relax and then circle around the other way. Breathe as normally as possible. Repeat this exercise in both directions, each twice.

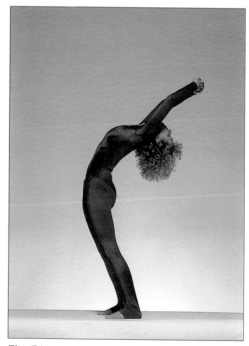

Fig. 31

III. This is the right way

Pull your buttocks together when
bending to the side to achieve even
more effect.
Leave your knees stretched out and do
not move the feet. The warrior is an
excellent exercise for those who want
to lose weight in one particular place.
During the stretching there is a
wonderful relaxed feeling.

Variations

1. Do the exercise exactly as described
   above, but standing on your toes.
2. Do the exercise without remaining
   in the position, but in a complete
   slow movement.
3. Enlarge the circle to include the
   whole body.

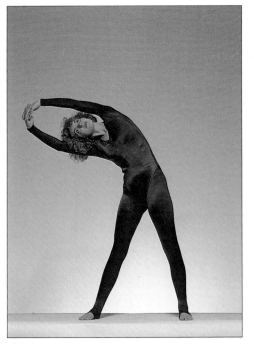

Fig. 32

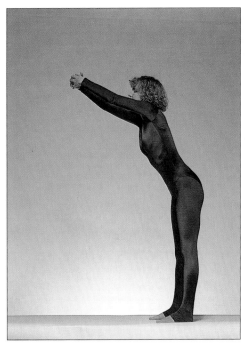

Fig. 33

Chest expander (Parsvottanasana)

I. What the exercise is good for

The chest expander
- develops the chest
- relieves tension in the neck, the shoulders and the upper part of the back
- creates new energy
- relaxes the whole body
- tightens the stomach muscles
- improves posture
- stretches the lungs and encourages a better blood circulation throughout the body

II. How to do it

1. Stand upright with legs slightly apart, arms forward, at shoulder height, palms on top of each other (Fig. 34).
2. Bring the arms round to the back with a wide sweeping movement, pull the shoulder blades together and fold the hands.
3. Push the pelvis forwards and, lifting the breast bone, stretch backwards gently.
4. Press your folded hands in the direction of your head and stay like this for 5 seconds (Fig. 35).
5. From this position, bend yourself forwards, lifting and bending from the hips. Let the weight of your body pull you downwards. Do not make any sudden movements (Fig. 36).
6. Stay in this position for 10 seconds and try at the same time to bring your hands further downwards to the head (Fig. 37, advanced position).
7. Bring yourself slowly upright again, relax, and repeat the exercise twice.

III. This is the right way

Repeat this exercise when you want to do something about your breasts.
Do not close your eyes while doing this exercise, as you will then find it easier to keep your balance.
The chest expander is a wonderful exercise that will liven you up if you have been sitting for hours at an office desk and feel tense and lifeless.

Caution. Taking the neck back (Fig. 35) can cause problems. Only do this exercise if your neck is supple.

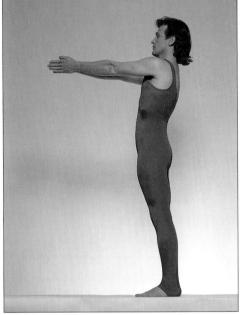

Fig. 34

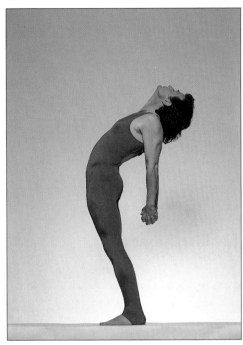

Fig. 35

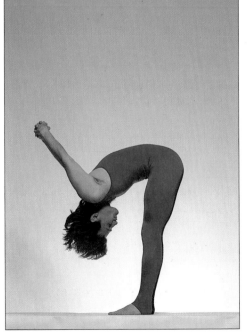

Fig. 36

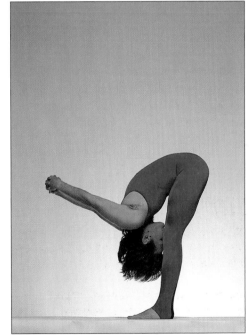

Fig. 37

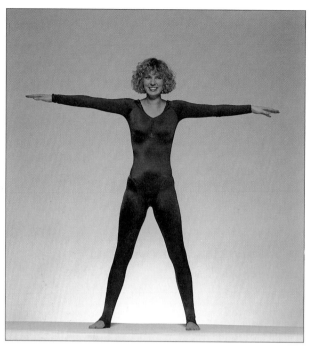

Fig. 38

Triangle (Trikonasana)

I. What the exercise is good for

The Triangle
- reduces back pain
- expands the chest
- relieves menstrual problems
- strengthens the thigh and upper and lower leg muscles
- massages the abdominal organs and encourages their functioning

II. How to do it

1. Stand with your legs apart. The distance should be about 1 yard (1 metre).
2. Stretch out your arms sideways, parallel to the floor (Fig. 38).
3. Turn your right foot 90 degrees outwards, the left foot slightly to the left.
4. Bend your body to the right side. Grasp the outside of your right leg with the right hand as far downwards as possible.
5. Lift up the left arm until it makes a straight line with the right. Look upwards to your left hand (Fig. 39).
6. Stay in this position for 10-30 seconds. Breathe as normally as possible.

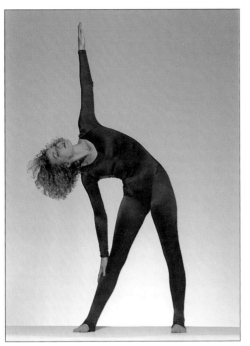

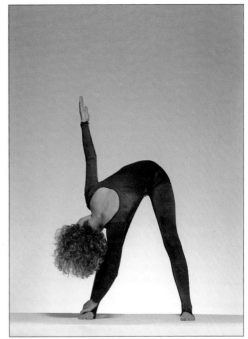

Fig. 39   Fig. 40

7. Straighten yourself out slowly.
8. Repeat the exercise on the other side.
9. Repeat the exercise twice on each side.

III. **This is the right way**

At all times the knees should be held completely straight. How far you come is not as critically important as doing the exercise properly.
Stretch your shoulders while remaining in the position.
The triangle resembles very much a gymnastic exercise that you probably know. It is remaining in position that has the effect of relieving tension. Try out both exercises, then you will be able to establish the difference.

Variation
1. Carry out steps 1 to 3 as described above.
2. Turn your body with outstretched arms to the right and guide your left arm as far as possible to the outside of the right foot.
3. Lift up the right arm high enough so that it forms a straight line with the left. Look upwards to your right hand (Fig. 40).
4. Steps 6, 7, 8 and 9 as described above.

Elbow swing

I. What the exercise is good for

The elbow swing
- ▶ relieves rheumatism and inflamed joints
- ▶ is relaxing
- ▶ keeps the arms supple

II. How to do it

1. Sit comfortably in the 'tailor' position, or sit upright.
2. Bend your elbows and lift them to shoulder height. Form the hands into a loose fist (Fig. 41).
3. Let your elbows rest by moving them suddenly forwards (Fig. 42).
4. Relax for a moment and repeat the exercise five times.

III. This is the right way

Make sure that the arms move properly suddenly forwards as though you were about to throw away your hands.
Yoga is concerned with every part of the body, even if this does not seem important – every one of them can be relaxed.
This exercise has the purpose of making your elbows move as though well greased (so that they do not creak and crack).

Caution. To avoid pain in the elbow, do not carry out this exercise too rapidly.

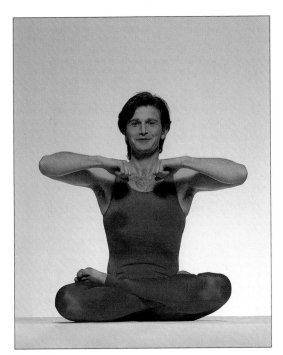

Fig. 41

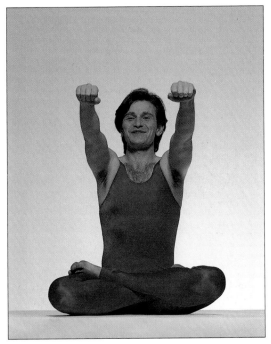

Fig. 42

Fish (Matsyasana)

I.   What the exercise is good for

The Fish
- ▶ is good for people with asthma and other breathing difficulties
- ▶ stimulates the thyroid gland and assists weight control
- ▶ loosens up and relaxes the neck region and the upper part of the back
- ▶ develops the chest and the breasts
- ▶ stimulates the digestion
- ▶ alleviates haemorrhoids
- ▶ encourages the blood circulation of the head

II.   How to do it

1. Lie down on the floor with outstretched legs. Place the palms of your hands downwards, half under the bottom. The elbows are slightly bent (Fig. 43).
2. Move the weight onto the elbows and lift up your chest by making a hollow. in the back.
3. At the same time bend the head back until you rest firmly on the floor with the vertex, or as far as you can (Fig. 44).
4. Now move your weight in such a way that most of the weight is carried by the bottom and elbows. There should be very little weight on the head.
5. Stay as long as you can (5–60 seconds) or until it becomes uncomfortable. Breathe as normally as possible.
6. Only come slowly out of the position, and repeat the exercise twice.

III.   This is the right way

Take care that your weight is carried largely on the bottom and the elbows. The legs must remain stretched out.
The Fish is an exercise of great therapeutic value for everyone who suffers with breathing difficulties as it relieves breathing due to the completely straight windpipe. Besides this, it helps to prevent tension in the neck region.
Do this exercise often and always after the Candle (page 66) and the Plough (page 90).

Caution. Avoid carrying out this exercise during menstruation, and also if you have an abdominal hernia or suffer from neck pain or vertigo.

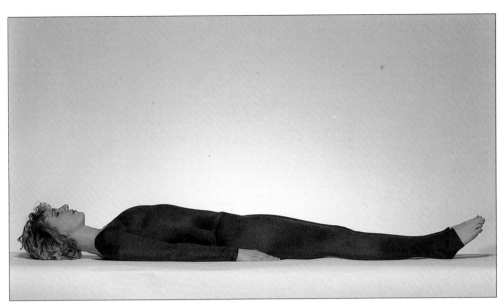

Fig. 43

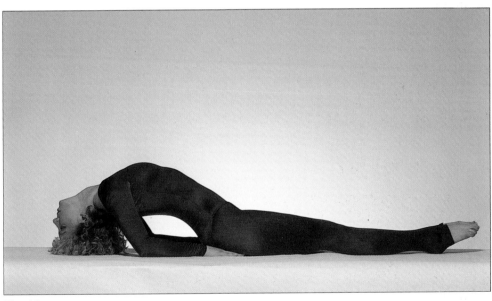

Fig. 44

51

Spread-leg stretching (Upavistha Konasana)

I. What the exercise is good for

The spread-leg stretching
- stretches and firms the leg tendons
- relaxes the whole body
- promotes good blood circulation in the whole pelvic region
- relieves pain caused by gout
- helps especially women, makes menstruation regular and encourages the functioning of the ovaries
- tightens the thighs and removes flab
- makes the spine supple and flexible

II. How to do it

1. Sit down with the legs wide apart and stretched out in front on the floor (Fig. 45).
2. Sitting tall, place your hands on the legs and let them slide gradually towards the toes. The legs remain stretched out.
3. Bend yourself from the waist forwards, a vertebra at a time. Then grasp with the hands the part of the leg that you can reach with ease (Fig. 46). Do not look down until you reach the final position.
4. Let your head fall forwards and bend your elbows upwards in order to stretch the spine more easily. Stay in this position for 10–30 seconds. Relax and come slowly out of the position.
5. Repeat the exercise twice.

III. This is the right way

Sit yourself comfortably on your pelvis, not your coccyx.
Hold your knees straight the whole time, otherwise the exercise will lose much of its effectiveness.
Do not make any sudden movements.
In the advanced form of this position (see Fig. 47) you can touch the floor with your head.
The exercise is particularly suitable for women, and should be done every day.

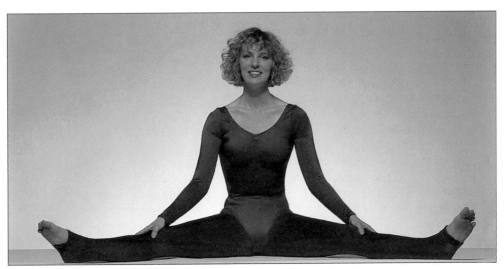

Fig. 45

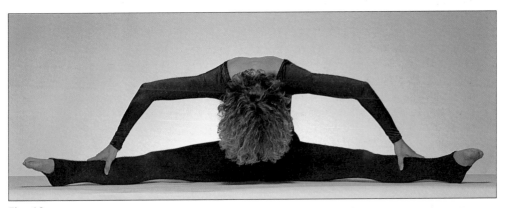

Fig. 46

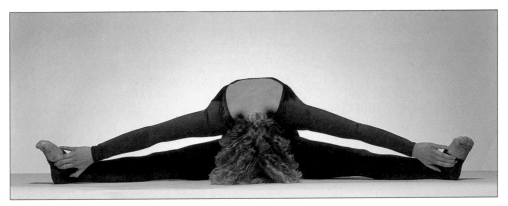

Fig. 47

Posture grip (Mukhasana variation)

I. What the exercise is good for

The posture grip
- alleviates mucus membrane infection and tense shoulders
- improves the posture, helps hanging shoulders
- builds and strengthens the upper arms
- trains the muscles around shoulder blades and upper part of the back
- lubricates the shoulder joints

II. How to do it

1. Sit comfortably with a straight back in the Japanese position (see Fig. 56).
2. Place your left hand on the back, the palm outwards and try to push it as far as you can up the back.
3. Stretch out your right hand, bend the elbow and lead your left hand to the spine. If your fingers are too wide apart from each other, then take a handkerchief between them (Fig. 49).
4. Now try to bring your hands together. Push them centimetre by centimetre together until the fingers touch and can grasp each other.
5. Stay in this position for 10–30 seconds. Try with the right hand to make a slight downwards movement and with the left an outward one. Or bend your body forwards until the head touches the knee (Figs. 50 and 51).
6. Repeat the exercise with the other hand, then another two per side.
7. Concentrate on the side on which you are most stiff.

III. This is the right way

Hold your back completely straight to increase the effectiveness of the exercise.
Do not overdo it. Only go as far as you can without it being painful.
The posture grip is an excellent exercise for freeing you from tension, especially if you have to spend a lot of time at an office desk. It evens out bad posture, which in turn has a very positive effect on your health.

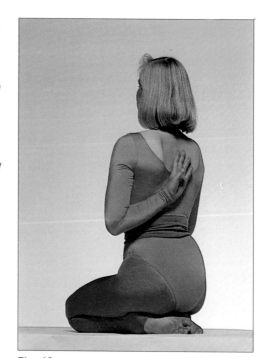

Fig. 48

54

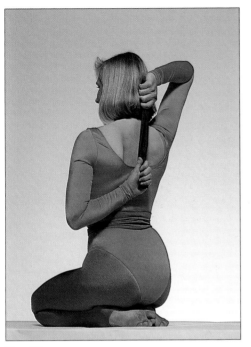

Fig. 49

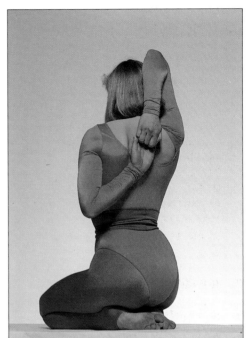

Fig. 50

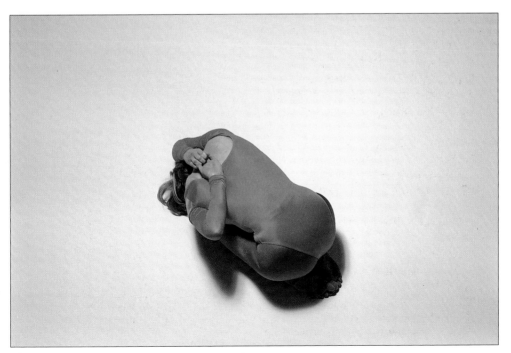

Fig. 51

Hands-on-the-wall exercise

I. What the exercise is good for

The hands-on-the-wall exercise
- firms and shapes the chest muscles
- develops the breasts
- strengthens arms and hand joints
- helps tense shoulders

II. How to do it

1. Stand up straight with the face to the wall.
2. Place the palms of your hands against the wall so that the fingertips point to each other and lightly touch.
3. Move yourself an arm's length from the wall (Fig. 52).
4. Slowly bend the elbows, the body remaining quite straight.
5. Press yourself now – more with the palms of the hand than the whole hand – against the wall, and create a contrary pressure to your body, which will quite slowly draw near to the wall. Slowly bring your forehead to the wall. Be careful that you do not bend at the waist and stick out your bottom — your body should form a completely straight line (Fig. 53).
6. Remain in this position for 5–15 seconds, and then press yourself back with the palms of your hand.
7. Relax.

III. This is the right way

Be careful that your body is kept in a straight line from the shoulders to the feet when pressing yourself at arm's length from the wall.

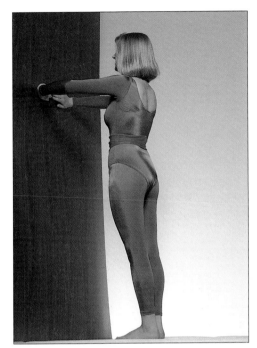

Fig. 52

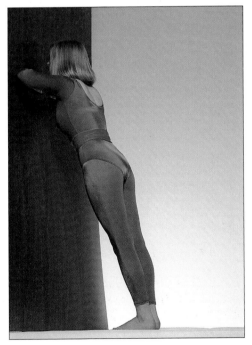

Fig. 53

Locust (Salabhasana)

I. What the exercise is good for

The Locust
- helps a slipped disc
- tightens the bottom
- removes flab from the hips
- encourages digestion
- has a good effect on the bladder
- stretches the spine and makes it supple
- relieves pain in the back, sacrum, lumbar region
- firms the stomach muscles

II. How to do it

1. Lie on your stomach on the ground. The arms are stretched out in front (Fig. 54).
2. Pull the buttocks together and press the sacrum down. Slowly lift, and all at the same time, the head, chest and legs as high as they will go without straining the back.
3. Balance on the lower abdomen. Stay in this position as long as you can. Breathe as normally as possible.
4. Repeat the exercise twice.

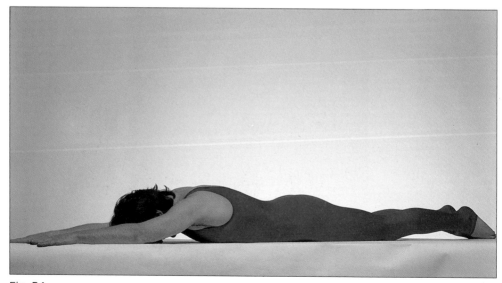

Fig. 54

58

III. This is the right way

Keep the legs closed for a greater effect.
If you want to strengthen the muscles of the upper back, you must not support yourself on your hands.
Do not become discouraged if the legs and the chest only just leave the ground. That becomes better little by little.

Caution. Avoid this posture if you have high blood pressure or a heart disorder.

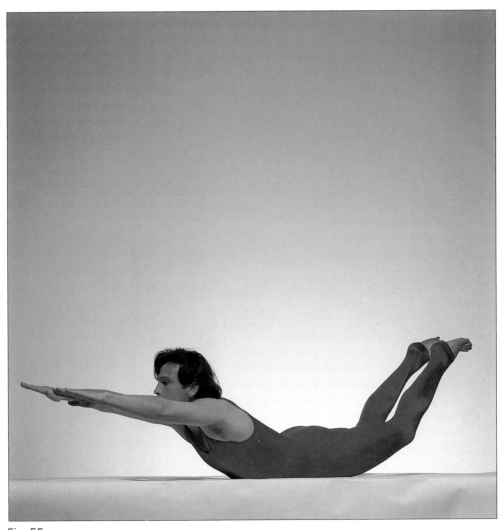

Fig. 55

Japanese (Diamond) sitting position (Virasana variation)

I. What the exercise is good for

The Japanese sitting position
- relieves tense ankles
- stretches the upper side of the leg
- makes the knee joints supple
- does a lot of good to varicose veins and tired legs
- relaxes the whole foot, especially the instep

II. How to do it

1. Kneel down upright with feet together, pointing the tips of the toes backwards.
2. Sit down slowly with your bottom on your heels. You can, if you wish, support yourself with your hands.
3. Relax by placing your whole weight on your heels. Keep your back completely straight all the time (Fig. 56).
4. If you find the exercise easy to do, let the heels fall apart, letting the toes point to each other and then try to sit in this 'nest'.

III. This is the right way

Sit down as often as possible. Always make sure that your back is quite straight. The floor is your exercise place.

Always prefer the floor to your so-called comfortable easy-chair, thus avoiding a deterioration of your posture.

Once you have overcome initial stiffness (this will go quicker than you think), this exercise will have a most beneficial effect on your nerves and muscles.

Caution. Avoid this posture if you have venous blood clots in your legs.

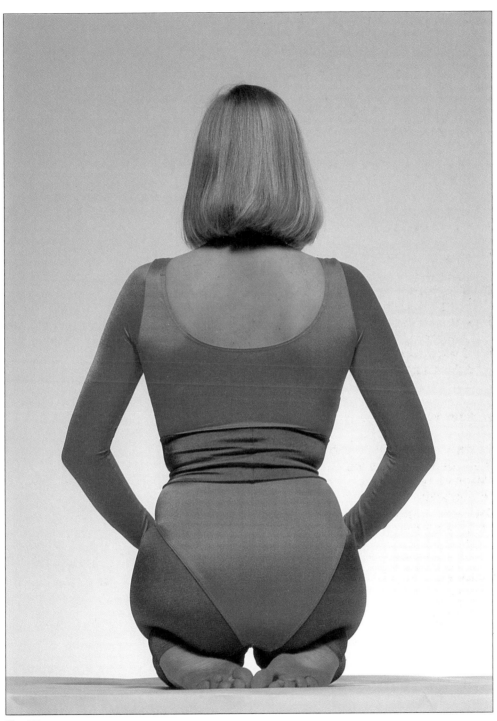

61

Fig. 56

Camel (Usthrasana)

I. What the exercise is good for

The Camel
- ▶ makes the spine supple and strengthens it
- ▶ provides energy and improves posture
- ▶ has a positive effect on round shoulders

II. How to do it

1. Kneel down upright, legs a little apart and toes pointing backwards. Place your hands on the back of your hips and let your head fall backwards (Fig. 57).
2. Move your pelvis forwards and downwards while lifting your breast bone as high as you can.
3. Hang the right hand over the right heel and the left hand over the left heel. If you can, place the palms of the hands on the soles of the feet (Fig. 58).
4. Pull in the buttocks and stretch the thighs and pelvis forwards as far as possible (Fig. 59). Stay in this position as long as possible. Breathe normally.
5. Repeat the exercise twice.

III. This is the right way

Concentrate as much as possible on stretching the chest and pelvis forwards (it will then be much easier to bend backwards).

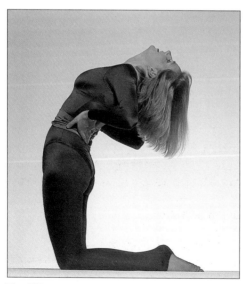

Fig. 57

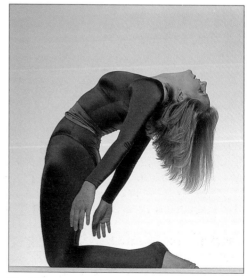

Fig. 58

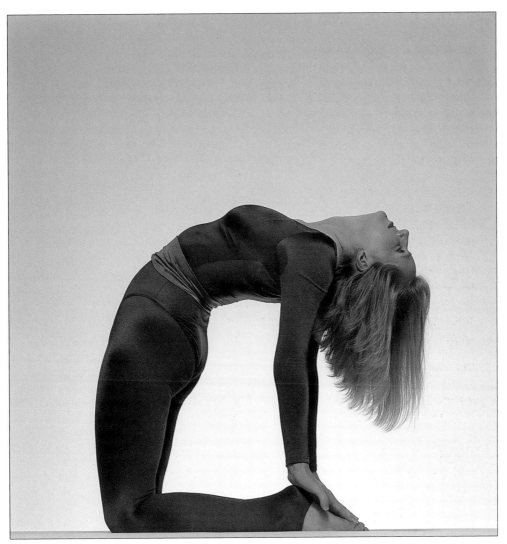

Fig. 59

Only bend as far backwards as you can without effort or pain.
At the beginning in this exercise you can leave your hands to fall where they will. Do not be too concerned if you are not able to touch your feet. This asana is gentle and is very good for the spine.
The stretching of the pelvis is a logical closing exercise.

Caution. This is a more advanced exercise and must be approached with caution. Also avoid this exercise if you have heart trouble, high blood pressure or a hernia, and also if you suffer from neck pain or spinal disc problems. Do not perform it in pregnancy or menstruation.

Cat stretching

I. What the exercise is good for

Cat stretching
- strengthens the back
- aids relaxation
- is suitable for women who have just given birth (it firms flabby organs)
- tightens the chin area
- stretches the whole of the front of the body
- strengthens the arms

II. How to do it

1. Kneel down on all fours.
2. Roll yourself lightly backwards (Fig. 60). Move your chest forwards and downwards as though you were trying to sweep the floor with it. Try to rest your Adam's apple on the ground (Fig. 61).
3. Stay like this for 5 seconds. All your weight should be resting on your arms.
4. Now return to the starting position and arch your back nicely (Fig. 62).
5. Stay like this for 5 seconds and then relax.
6. Move your right knee now in the direction of your head, trying to touch it. Stay like this for 5 seconds (Fig. 63).
7. Now stretch your right leg up backwards, keeping it perfectly straight. Stay like this with the head raised and the arms outstretched (Fig. 64).
8. Bring your leg quite slowly back to the head, and stay in this position.
9. Relax and repeat the exercise with the other leg.
10. Repeat the whole exercise once more (twice, if you like).

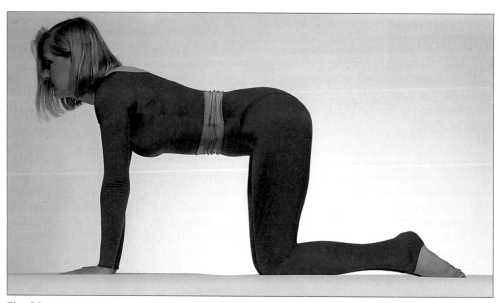

Fig. 60

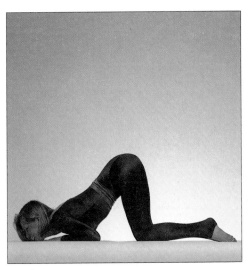

Fig. 61

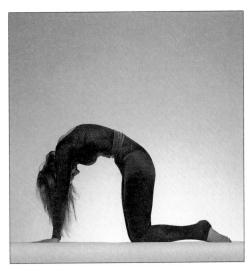

Fig. 62

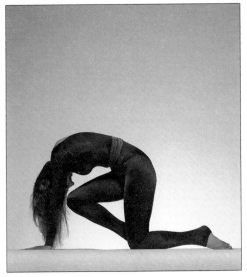

Fig. 63

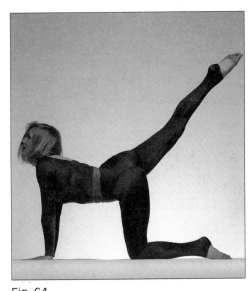

Fig. 64

III. This is the right way

Be happy about the way your body stretches out. Move yourself slowly and gracefully. Do not become discouraged if you cannot bring your knee right up to the head.

Cat stretching is recommended by gynaecologists after childbirth. It relieves pain in the lower back and stomach region.

Caution. Avoid this exercise if you suffer from epilepsy.

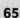

Candle (Sarvangasana)

I. What the exercise is good for

The Candle
- has a positive effect on the whole organism
- promotes a good circulation of blood through the brain, the spine and the pelvic region (as a result of our upright posture, normally insufficient blood containing oxygen reaches these)
- strengthens and balances the central nervous system (prevents stress and sleeplessness)
- stimulates the functioning of the endocrine glands
- relieves palpitations, shortness of breath, bronchitis, coughing, and asthma in the chest and neck region by increasing blood circulation
- because of the upside-down position the abdominal organs are relieved of their opposing pressure on each other, which encourages digestion, frees the body of poisons and brings new energy and vitality
- is a help in cases of menstrual problems and haemorrhoids
- relieves varicose veins
- brings life to the lethargic and anaemic
- relaxes the whole body
- stimulates the sex glands and organs
- stretches the spine
- strengthens and firms the back, leg, neck and stomach muscles

II. How to do it

1. Lie down on a thick blanket with your legs stretched out. The hands should be placed palms down close to the sides of the body.
2. Draw in the lower abdominal muscles and bend your knees to your chest. Lift the legs slowly until they are at right angles to the floor.

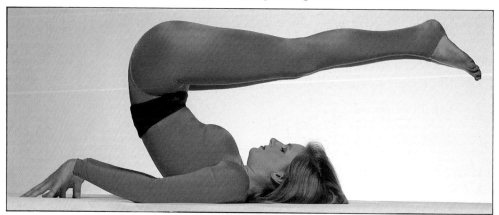

Fig. 65

3. Support yourself on your fingertips (Fig. 65).
4. Lift up your bottom and the lower part of the back. Now support yourself at the waist with the hands, the thumbs towards the stomach. The *elbows must stay close to the body* (Fig. 66).
5. Stretch your legs out as straight as a candle and pull in your bottom as far as your balance will allow.
6. As soon as you have finished balancing, support yourself with the hands further up at the ribs, and pull the bottom in still further (Fig. 67).
7. Stretch out your legs and tips of the toes as far as you can. As a beginner, just stay in this position for 10–60 seconds. Increase this slowly up to 3 minutes. Breathe normally during the exercise.
8. When you are ready to come out of the posture, bend your knees towards your forehead and roll slowly out of the position, pulling in your lower abdominal muscles, until your hips rest on the floor. Remain with knees to chest for a few breaths before slowly stretching the legs out.

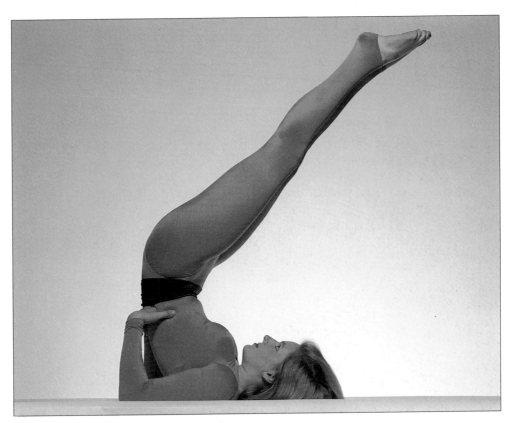

Fig. 66

III. This is the right way

Have some patience. The most important thing is that you stretch out upwards, even if you are not quite straight.
At first you may feel a little dizzy. This is quite normal and it is because the veins suddenly widen.

Caution. Do not practise the Candle during menstruation. Omit this exercise if you suffer from back pain, heart disease, or if your blood pressure is too high or too low. If in doubt, consult your doctor.

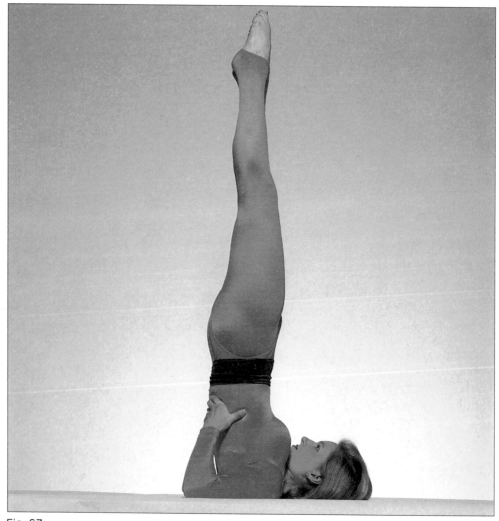

Fig. 67

Bell

I. What the exercise is good for

The Bell
▶ relieves problems in the shoulders and joints
▶ firms the chest muscles
▶ helps against tension in the shoulders and upper back

How to do it

1. Sit comfortably in the 'tailor' position.
2. Bend the elbows and lift them to shoulder level so that the tips of the fingers touch (Fig. 68).
3. Push your shoulder blades so close together that you can almost hold a banknote between them. Hold the elbows as high as you can.
4. Stay like this for 5–10 seconds (Fig. 69).
5. Come slowly out of this position and then shrug the shoulders.
6. Repeat the exercise three to five times. in this way you will achieve the optimum effect.

III. This is the right way

Loosen all tense muscles by shrugging the shoulders. Usually the shoulders are initially braced and usually the loosening of the tension is first really felt there. When bringing the shoulder blades together, you must not lift up the shoulders. And try at all costs to keep the elbows up high.

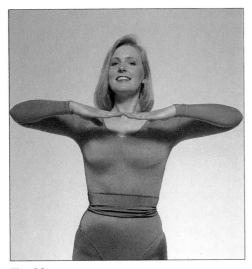

Fig. 68

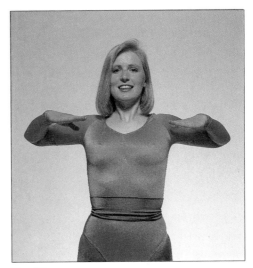

Fig. 69

69

Knee and leg stretching (Baddha Konasana)

I. What the exercise is good for

Knee and leg stretching
 ▶ relieves bladder problems
 ▶ keeps the prostate gland healthy
 ▶ stimulates the kidneys
 ▶ firms the inner side of the upper leg
 ▶ livens up tired legs
 ▶ helps women in preparation for childbirth
 ▶ stimulates the functioning of the ovaries and ensures regular menstruation
 ▶ relieves sciatica pain

How to do it

1. Sit yourself on the floor with outstretched legs and a straight back.
2. Bend the knees to the side and place the soles of the feet against each other (Fig. 70).
3. Hold the toes tightly, and pull the feet as far as possible towards the body – if you can, as far as the crotch (Fig 71).
4. Using great determination spread open the legs and by pulling try to get the knee onto the floor.
5. Stay in this position for 5–30 seconds. Breathe normally all the time (Fig. 72).
6. Relax by stretching out the legs again. You can also shake them, as you wish.
7. Repeat the exercise twice. If you really want to do something for your health and fight the flabby insides of your thighs, then do the exercise four times or more.

III. This is the right way

Hold your toes quite firmly so that you do not slip.
Do not press your knees downwards by force. You will achieve far more by force of will. Do not become discouraged if at the beginning your knees stick up like peaks. Given sufficient patience success will eventually be yours. Try to relax completely, even when remaining in the position. Stretching legs and knees is tiring but important. Medical experiments have shown that Indian shoemakers, from whom this position has been copied, hardly ever suffer bladder problems.

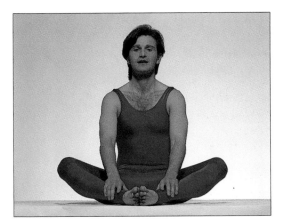

Fig. 70

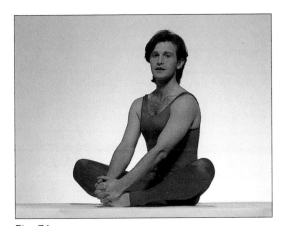

Fig. 71

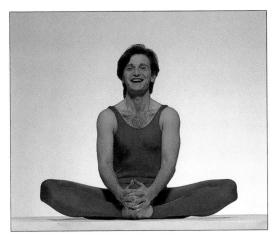

Fig. 72

Ankle bending

I. What the exercise is good for

Ankle bending
▶ helps to prevent swollen ankles and feet
▶ strengthens weak ankles
▶ encourages the blood circulation and livens up tired legs
▶ shapes legs and ankles

II. How to do it

1. Stand up straight with the feet a few centimetres apart.
2. Roll your feet to the right. This means you will be standing on the right outer side of your right foot and the right inner side of your left foot (Fig. 73).
3. Now bend your knee to the right and forwards, at the same time keeping your pelvis and thighs straight.
4. Stay like this for 5 seconds, or until you feel uncomfortable.
5. Do the same on the other side.
6. First lift the one foot from the floor, the tips of the toes towards the front, and rotate it first clockwise and then anti-clockwise (Fig. 74).
7. Do the same with the other foot.
8. Repeat these two exercises twice more.

III. This is the right way

If you do this exercise regularly, it will put a youthful spring in your step. Stiff ankles are the first sign of ageing.
Please make sure that your pelvis points forwards without moving and does not bend to the right or to the left. The whole exercise will then prove to be very effective.

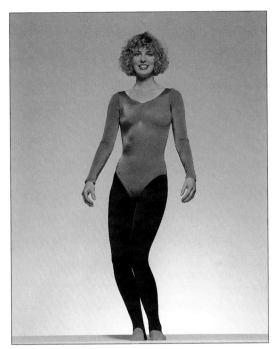

Fig. 73

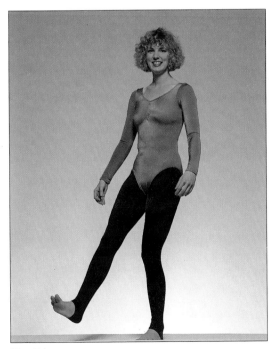

Fig. 74

Cobra (Bhujangasana)

I. What the exercise is good for

The Cobra
- develops the chest muscles
- stretches and compresses the spine, helps to prevent spine damage
- strengthens the stomach and back muscles
- firms the buttocks and reduces flab
- strengthens the nervous system
- promotes digestion
- alleviates abdominal troubles
- firms the chin region

II. How to do it

1. Lie down on your stomach with your hands palm downwards under your shoulders (Fig. 75).
2. Lift your head slightly from the floor and move your chest forwards.
3. Pressing down with your thighs and using your back muscles, begin to raise your trunk from the floor.
4. Take the weight with your hands and roll your shoulders back and down, moving your chest forward like the hood of a cobra.
5. Look straight ahead and keep your pubic bone in contact with the mat (Fig. 76). Do not let your head fall too far back.
6. Stay in this position taking rhythmic breaths until it becomes uncomfortable (5–30 seconds).
7. Come out of the Cobra very slowly, transferring your weight from your hands to your back muscles as soon as you can.
8. Repeat the exercise twice, and breathe as normally as possible.

III. This is the right way

When going into this position remember to do most of the work with the back muscles. The hands are used for support in the final stages only. Keep looking forward until you have fully extended your spine – you can then take your head back to look up at the ceiling if you like. Try to experience consciously the slow movement of your spine and enjoy it as though someone were massaging it.

Caution. Avoid practising this exercise in pregnancy, or if you have a hernia.

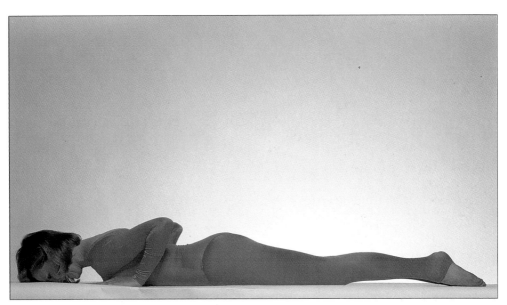

Fig. 75

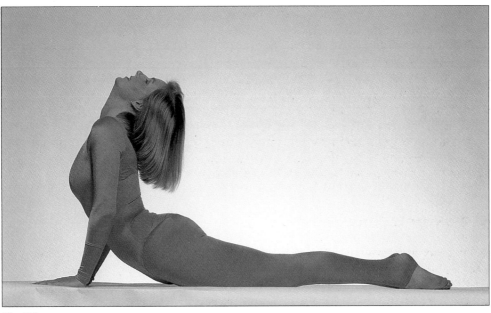

Fig. 76

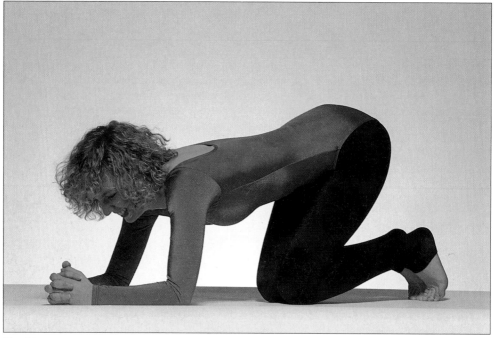

Fig. 77

Headstand (Salamba Shirshasana)

This is an excellent exercise although not an easy one, so practise your simpler yoga positions first before moving on to the exercise.

I. What the exercise is good for

The headstand
- ▶ stimulates blood circulation; this is particularly good for those parts of the body where circulation is normally bad, such as the brain, heart, pelvis and spine.
- ▶ strengthens the nervous system
- ▶ puts the abdominal organs back into their proper position
- ▶ firms and strengthens the stomach muscles
- ▶ stimulates the endocrine glands
- ▶ strengthens the lungs
- ▶ brings new energy and vitality
- ▶ alleviates problems such as sleeplessness, nervous tension, colds, sore throat, palpitations, asthma, and a lot more.

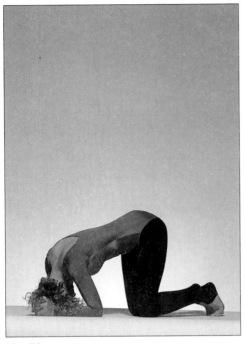

Fig. 78

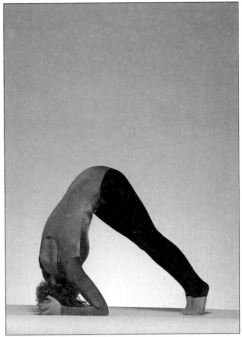

Fig. 79

ii. How to do it

1. Make sure that you have something suitable on the floor for your head to rest on, either a carpet or a blanket folded several times.
2. Kneel on the carpet or in front of the blanket with your bottom resting on your heels.
3. Fold the hands and lay them on the floor with the elbows a shoulder-width apart (Fig. 77).
4. Place your head on the floor so that the whole of the forehead is touching the floor. Do not worry about your hands at this point.
5. Now pull the folded hands to the head so that the little fingers are wedged under the curvature of the skull (Fig. 78).
6. Lift up your bottom, bring your knees forward a little, and make a few steps on tiptoe towards the head. Keep the back straight (Fig. 79).
7. When you can go no further, stay in this position until it becomes uncomfortable. Then return slowly to the position you had at the start.
8. Relax and let your head hang down for a few moments.
9. Repeat twice more in order to develop a sense of balance (Figs 80, 81 and 82 show advanced positions).

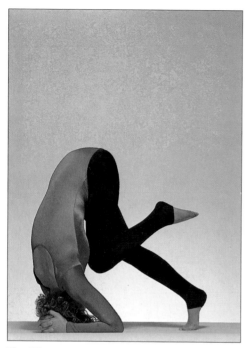

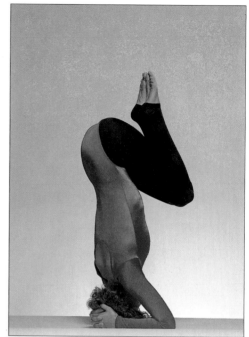

Fig. 80

Fig. 81

III. This is the right way

Fold your hands quite firmly. Be careful that your elbows do not separate or press against the head. In order to be an effective support they must be exactly a shoulder-width apart.

It is the centre of the head, the vertex, that must be placed on the floor. The time will come when you will be able to stand on your head for 5–30 minutes. Do not lead the head to the hands, but bring the folded hands to the head. Try it out until you have produced a comfortable 'nest' for your head.

Never push yourself off the floor with the tips of your toes. Only when the toes have almost automatically left the floor on their own can you bring up your legs. When you see that you are able to do it, test out the safety of your balance by first pressing the knee for a time onto your chest. The most difficult part of a proper headstand is bringing up the legs, which demands strong leg muscles. The headstand demands more strength than skill. First prepare yourself for the headstand, especially if you have round shoulders, by going into the Cobra (page 74) and the Bow (page 40). This will strengthen the neck muscles and make them flexible. If you find that at the moment you lift your legs you fall over, then practise pulling in the stomach to strengthen the stomach muscles. The headstand is one of the more difficult yoga positions. In order to do it, time is required and also strength, suppleness and an acute sense of balance. Develop these skills.

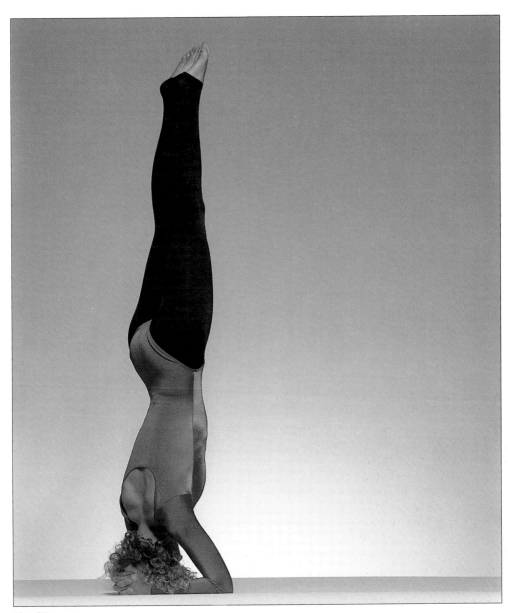

Fig. 82

Caution. Avoid this posture during menstruation. Omit it also if you have neck problems, postural defects, heart trouble or high blood pressure.

Head to knee stretching (Janu Shirshasana)

I. What the exercise is good for

Head to knee stretching
- strengthens and firms the stomach and legs
- minimises tension in the legs, in buttocks and back
- massages the abdominal organs and encourages their functioning
- strengthens the spine and makes it elastic

II. How to do it

1. Sit down keeping your back straight and stretch out your legs on the floor.
2. Bend the left leg, and bring the left foot (the knee stays on the floor) as near as possible to your body (Fig. 83).
3. Stretch out your arms and let them slide *slowly* down to your legs as far as you can. While doing this, stretch your upper body forwards (Fig. 84).
4. Hold yourself firm by the leg. Depending on how supple you are, that can be at the height of the knee, ankle or calf.
5. Bend your elbows outwards and downwards and extend yourself quite gently forwards and downwards. To avoid pulling a muscle, this must be done gently and without jerking.
6. Only go as far as you can without straining yourself and then stay in the position for 5–30 seconds. Breathe as normally as possible (Fig. 85).
7. Bring yourself up again slowly and repeat the exercise with the other leg.
8. Do this exercise three times on each side.

III. This is the right way

It is amazing what you can achieve with a little patience, bringing the head down to the knee or even below it. A stiff back and tense knee tendons are among the first signs of old age. This exercise releases both, even with arthritis. Try to keep the spine straight at all times and avoid pulling the head down to the knee.
Leave your knee on the floor and do not make any sudden or jerky movements. The benefit of this yoga exercise lies in remaining quite still while holding the position and this will prevent you from straining any muscle.

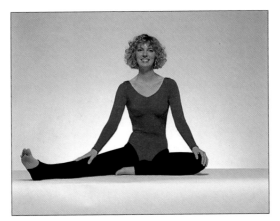

Fig. 83

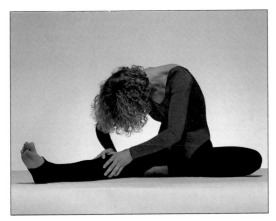

Fig. 84

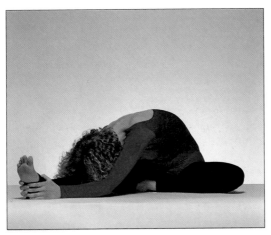

Fig. 85

Lion (Simhasana)

I. What the exercise is good for

The Lion
- relaxes the face
- firms the neck and face muscles
- reduces a double chin
- smooths out creases
- encourages blood circulation and makes the complexion fresh looking
- relieves sore throats and strengthens the voice

II. How to do it

1. Kneel down restfully with the bottom on the heels. The hands hang down onto the legs with the palms downwards (Fig. 86).
2. Spread your fingers and let them slowly slide forward until the fingertips touch the floor.
3. Bend your body forwards with the bottom off your heels, the arms stretched out.
4. Pull your eyes wide open.
5. Stick your tongue out as far as it will go. Try to touch your chin with your tongue (Fig. 87).
6. Stay in this position for 10 seconds.
7. Sit down again on the heels, pull in your tongue again and completely relax.
8. Repeat the exercise twice.

III. This is the right way

Stick your tongue right out.
Do not let yourself be irritated by the feeling of having a wooden handle in your mouth. This will only happen at the beginning and will later disappear.
Do this exercise with closed eyes facing the sun.
Enjoy the wonderful feeling of relaxation when you put your tongue back.
The Lion should be a must exercise for everyone. it is a natural beauty treatment, in smoothing folds and making the complexion fresher. Besides this, the exercise relieves tension – one can really work it off!

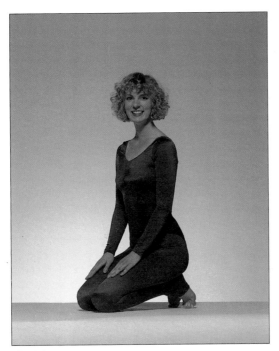

Fig. 86

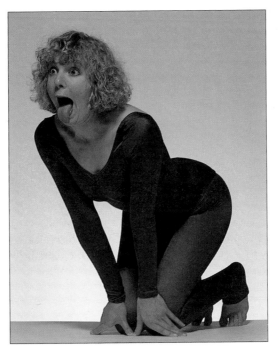

Fig. 87

Neck rolling

I. What the exercise is good for

Neck rolling
- helps in cases of deep-seated neck tension
- alleviates a stiff neck and often even headaches
- helps the whole body relax, especially in cases of sleeplessness
- reduces a double chin

II. How to do it

1. Sit down comfortably in the 'tailor' position or on a chair, with shoulders pulled back.
2. Let your head slowly tip forwards and hang like a lifeless puppet. Stay like that.
3. Lift your head again – keep the shoulders straight – and let it fall backwards. How far you will be able to do this will depend on how tense you are (Fig. 88).
4. Leaving your mouth firmly closed, stay like that.
5. Let your head fall to one side and then to the other. Look upwards while doing it and hold the position on each side for a few seconds (Figs 89 and 90).
6. Just imagine that you are a rag doll and let your head hang down. Roll in an unbroken gentle movement first to the right, then backwards, then left and forwards. This rolling should not be consciously controlled; it has to be a free, circling, loose moving of the head.
7. Repeat this circling in the other direction. Do the complete exercise another three times.

III. This is the right way

Rolling the neck is a unique exercise for relaxation and a quick refill of energy. Close your eyes while doing it and you will feel how the tension gradually recedes. Go through the exercise very slowly and carefully; let your head roll gently over the tense areas. At the beginning you may hear one or two cracking sounds, but they will soon disappear if you do the exercise regularly. The neck joints are lubricated as a result of this exercise. The feeling that neck and spine are welded together is one of the first signs of ageing.

Caution. Do not try to stretch your head too far back, to avoid future neck problems.

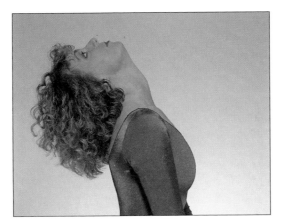

Fig. 88

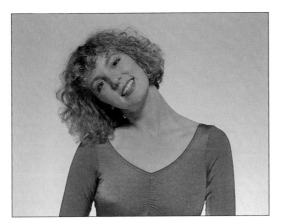

Fig. 89

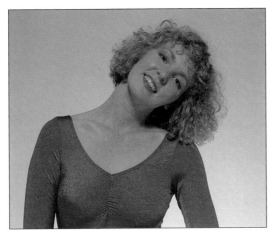

Fig. 90

Pendulum

I. What the exercise is good for

The Pendulum
- relieves pain in the shoulders
- encourages blood circulation in the head and upper parts of the body
- relieves tension and gives a feeling of energy
- improves posture
- strengthens the shoulder muscles and upper back

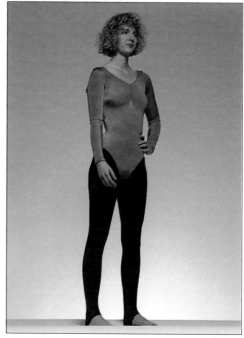

Fig. 91

II. How to do it

1. Stand comfortably with feet part and rest your left hand on the waist (Fig. 91).
2. Bend slowly forwards from the hips and let your right arm hang limply downwards.
3. Now swing the right arm in front of the legs like a pendulum, backwards and forwards. In doing this it is important that this is not controlled by your will. Your arm should move pendulum fashion as though on its own (Fig. 92).
4. Straighten yourself up again and put your right arm behind your head. Stretch it as far as it will go backwards. Stay like that, and then relax (Fig. 93).
5. Repeat the whole thing again with the other arm.
6. Repeat again but with both arms.
7. Repeat the whole thing two or three times and swing in both directions.

III. This is the right way

Keep the knees straight. Be careful not to swing your arm stiffly.
To those who have no real problems this exercise may appear deceptively simple. To those who are tense or have pain in the shoulders, this asana will bring great relief.

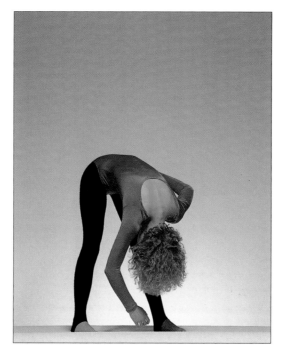

Fig. 92

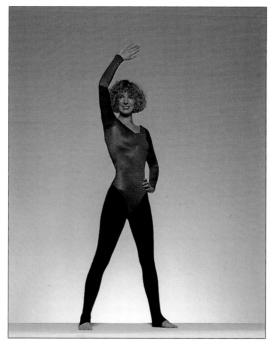

Fig. 93

Half-lotus (Ardha Padmasana)

I. What the exercise is good for

The Half-lotus
▶ is ideal for long periods of sitting
▶ relaxes the whole body
▶ stretches and strengthens the legs and the lower part of the body
▶ has a positive effect on the bladder and urinary tract

II. How to do it

1. Sit down on the floor with the legs spread and stretched out.
2. Bring the sole of the right foot in to the upper part of the left thigh. The right knee remains on the floor.
3. Bend the left leg, grasp the toes firmly with both hands, and place the left foot carefully on the right lower leg.
4. So that you do not become uncomfortable, preferably place the ankles side by side; if they lie one on top of the other it will hurt. Now bring the toes of the left foot in the cleft made by the upper leg and the calf of the right leg (Fig. 94).
5. Hold your back up completely straight. Both knees should remain as near as possible to each other on the floor.
6. Stay in this position until you become uncomfortable.
7. Repeat the exercise with the other leg.

III. This is the right way

As in the case of most yoga positions none of these should be forced. Force nothing. Some make this position straight off, some will take a year or longer. Because the muscles of the knee tend to be easily strained, wrongly directed ambition can cause damage. Do not give up, but try it again and again even if your knee is pointing up to the sky and will not remain on the floor. In the long term this position is very comfortable and above all healthy.

Caution. Omit this position if you have venous blood clots in your legs.

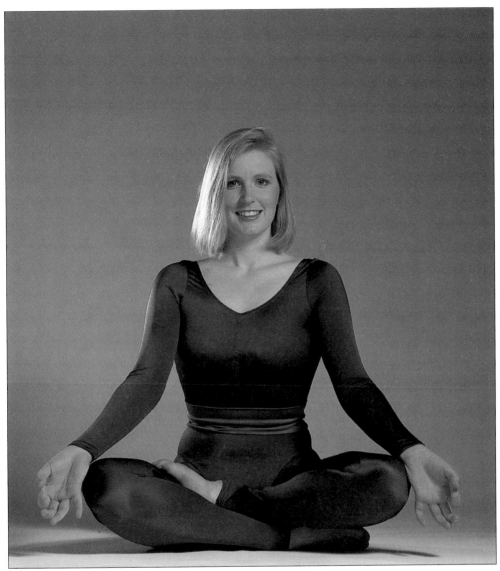

Fig. 94

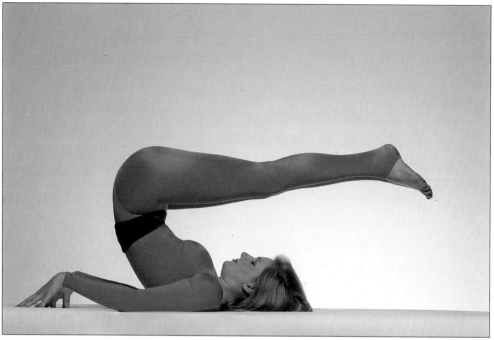

Fig. 95

Plough (Halasana)

I. What the exercise is good for

The Plough
- makes the spine elastic
- stimulates the thyroid gland
- strengthens and firms the muscles of the stomach
- tones the legs and hips and makes them slimmer
- relieves deep-seated tension and headaches
- strengthens the nervous system
- stimulates the blood circulation
- massages the spleen, liver, pancreas and kidneys
- encourages energy and vitality
- strengthens the neck
- helps to reduce large breasts

II. How to do it

1. Lie down on your back with outstretched legs, the arms lying at the side with the palms downwards.

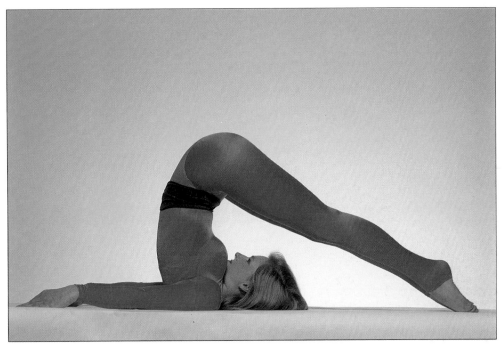

Fig. 96

2. Bend the knees, then lift up the legs by tensing the stomach and leg muscles.
3. Support yourself with the fingertips and in this way lift up the bottom and the lower part of the back (Fig. 95).
4. Push your legs over the head and try to touch the floor with your toes. To do this you will have to bend at the waist. Keep the knees straight (Fig. 96). If your feet do not reach the floor, rest them on a low stool.
5. Stay in that position as long as you are still comfortable (if possible for a minute).
6. Breathe normally.
7. Come out of the position slowly by drawing in the abdominal muscles and rolling the spine down to the mat with knees bent. When your hips are down, place your feet on the floor with knees still bent and rest for a moment before stretching out fully (Figs. 97 and 98 are advanced positions).

III. This is the right way

Do not become discouraged if you can only raise your bottom a few inches off the floor. Only go as far as you can, stay in that position and repeat it a few times. Staying in the position will already strengthen the muscles. Do not lift up

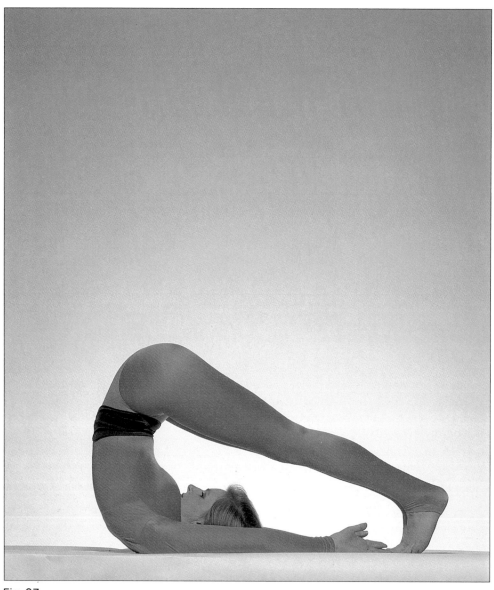

Fig. 97

your head if your bring your feet back onto the ground. Be careful that your knees are always straight.

Breathe as normally as possible. The more you practise the easier this exercise will become.

If you have a feeling of breathlessness, support your legs on a small stool behind you. You will be amazed at the quick progress you make with the Plough.

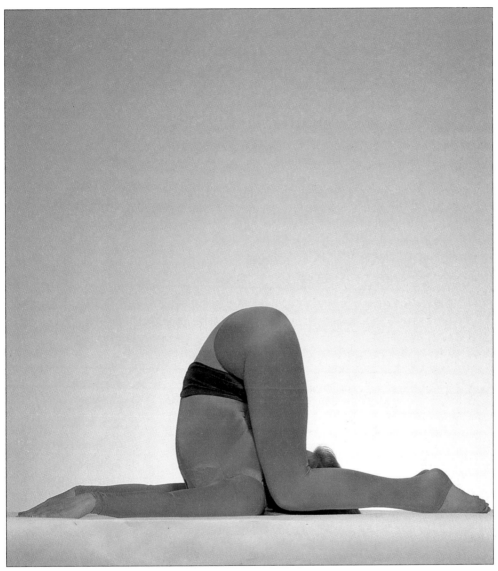

Fig. 98

Even older people will manage to get their toes onto the ground in a relatively short time. The spine is often unnaturally compressed after years of a false posture. This asana stretches and relaxes the whole body.

Caution. Do not practise the Plough during menstruation or in pregnancy. Omit it also if you have a hernia, uterine prolapse, hypertension, a spinal disc problem or neck pain.

Pump (Urdhva Prasarita Padasana)

This is a more advanced exercise and should only be attempted carefully by those with some experience.

I. What the exercise is good for

The Pump
- stimulates the blood circulation of the whole body
- firms and stretches the stomach and buttocks
- strengthens the back muscles
- removes flab around the waist
- strengthens and massages the abdominal organs
- alleviates flatulence, helps digestion

II. How to do it

1. Lie flat on your back. The arms lie with the palms downwards on the body, half under the bottom.
2. Press against the floor with your palms, with the legs stretched out and closed together.
3. Slowly raise your outstretched legs (Fig. 99). Then after 5–10 seconds you should form a right angle with the floor.
4. Remain in the position (Fig. 100).
5. Bring your legs down to the floor again – the nearer you are to the floor the slower this should be (Fig. 101).
6. Repeat the exercise several times.

III. This is the right way

In order to use the exercise to maximum effect, you must move yourself only slowly. The nearer the floor you are the slower you must be.
Leave the knee completely straight and stay with your head on the floor when you leave the position. To avoid straining the back or legs, you can bend the legs over the abdomen and then straighten them to a right angle.
Do not hold your breath.
The Pump is a must for strengthening the stomach muscles. It takes a lot of energy, but the results are always satisfying.

Caution. This is an advanced exercise. Omit this exercise during menstruation and in pregnancy. If you have weak stomach muscles or have recently given birth, do the exercise using one leg only at first.

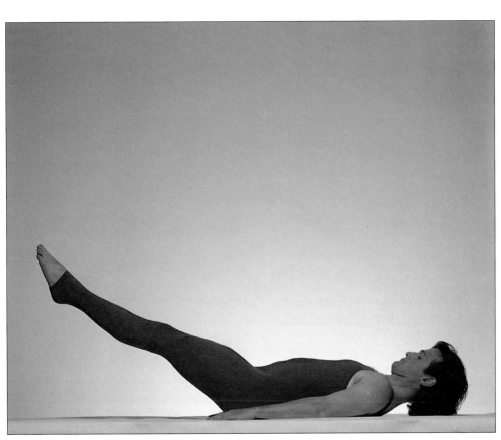

Fig. 99

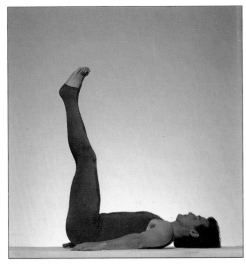

Fig. 100

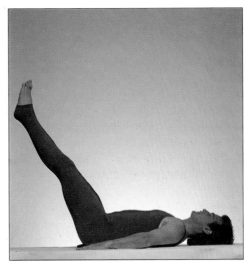

Fig. 101

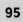

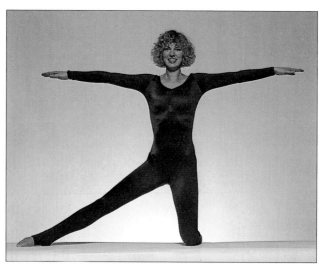
Fig. 102

Crossbars (Parighasana)

I. What the exercise is good for

Crossbars
- ▶ tightens the abdominal wall
- ▶ tightens and shapes the inside of the thigh
- ▶ relieves a stiff back
- ▶ stretches the whole pelvic region
- ▶ stimulates the lower abdominal organs
- ▶ trains the ankles

II. How to do it

1. Kneel up straight on the floor, the feet remaining together.
2. Stretch out the right leg to the right. Make certain that your knee and tips of the toes are stretched out.
3. Lift your arms sideways (Fig. 102).
4. Place the right arm with the palms upwards on the right leg.
5. Bend your body to the right, and let the right ear rest on the arm (Fig. 103).
6. Lift your left arm slowly above the head and try to bring it as far as the right hand so that the palms touch.
7. Look to the front all the time while opening the arms.
8. Remain like this as long as you can without strain (5–30 seconds), and breathe all the time as normally as possible.

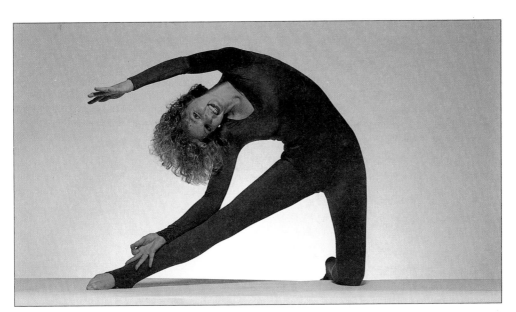

Fig. 103

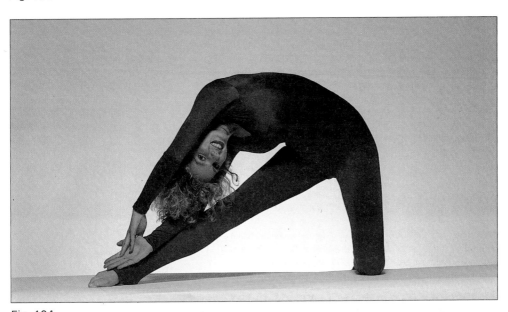

Fig. 104

III. This is the right way

Under no circumstances should you become discouraged if at the beginning you cannot reach the ideal position. The beauty of yoga is that each day you will make more progress.

Bend yourself from the waist not forwards, but sideways.

Rock 'n' roll

I. What the exercise is good for

Rock 'n' roll
- brings a feeling of warmth and energy
- makes the spine supple and pliable
- strengthens the stomach muscles
- massages and alleviates tension in the neck and along the spine
- stimulates the liver and the spleen
- encourages digestion and evacuation

II. How to do it

1. Sit on the floor with your legs drawn up.
2. Fold your hands below the knees.
3. Bring your head as near as possible to the knees and leave it there during the exercise (Fig. 105).
4. Gently roll backwards on your spine. Keep the back rounded and the feet together (Fig. 106).
5. Roll with a gentle rhythm backwards and forwards (Fig. 107).
6. Roll 12 times or for one minute.
7. Do not forget breathing: when rolling backwards breathe in, and when rolling forwards breathe out.

III. This is the right way

Begin this exercise from the lying position if you are a little afraid to begin with sitting.
Do this exercise whenever you feel tensed up.
Be careful during the whole exercise to keep your head as close as possible to your knees. This will make your back nice and round and you can then roll on it much better.
Use the backwards roll to gain momentum for the forwards roll. Do not land too heavily on your feet as you may jar your spine.
This exercise is a favourite of my husband, when he arrives home from the office in the evening completely shattered. Instead of slumping down motionless in front of the television, he does this exercise as soon as he gets home before his evening meal. He knows that it relaxes him and preserves what is left of the day.

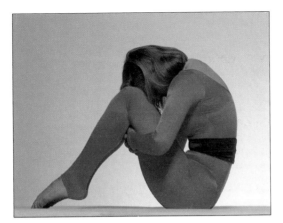

Fig. 105

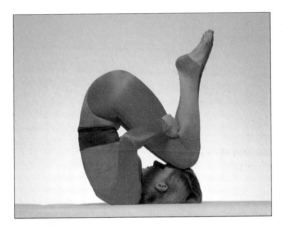

Fig. 106

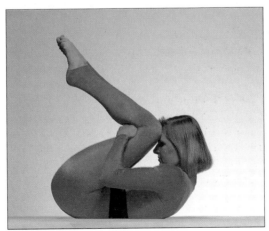

Fig. 107

Forward-bend sitting (Paschimottanasana)

I. What the exercise is good for

Forward-bend sitting
▶ strengthens the stomach muscles and the inner organs
▶ stretches and makes the legs and spine more pliable and supple
▶ strengthens the whole nervous system
▶ encourages digestion and evacuation
▶ strengthens the kidneys
▶ massages the heart
▶ stretches the pelvic area and ensures its circulation with blood
▶ gives a feeling of vitality

II. How to do it

1. Sit on the floor with legs closed and stretched out (Fig. 108). 'Walk' the buttocks back until your weight is 'sitting' on the bones.
2. Lift your arms above the head and stretch your spine looking straight ahead.
3. Roll forward from the hips, vertebra by vertebra, until you can grasp your feet, ankles or lower legs (Fig. 110).
4. Bend your elbows outwards and try to lengthen your body forwards and downwards.
5. Let your head hang forwards but do not try to pull it downwards to the legs. Stay in this position for 5–10 seconds and breathe the whole time as normally as possible (Fig. 111).
6. Straighten up very slowly and repeat the exercise twice.
7. With time it will be possible to place your head on your knees and to grasp the toes (instead of the ankles) by placing your elbows on the ground.

III. This is the right way

Stay all the time over your outstretched legs and remain totally immobile, otherwise you will waste time and have trouble.
Do not make any jerky movements in order to get further or deeper, as you can then cause painful strains.
It is far more important that a previously stiff and unbending spine be bent forwards rather than downwards. And yet, despite this, you will be surprised how quickly you make progress that previously you would not have thought possible!

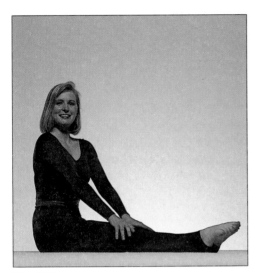

Fig. 108

Caution. Omit this exercise if you are pregnant, or if you have a hernia.

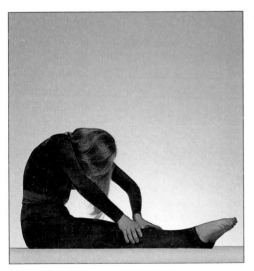

Fig. 110

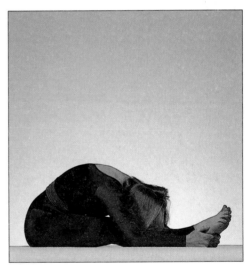

Fig. 111

Forward-bend standing (Padahastasana)

I. What the exercise is good for

Forward-bend standing
- helps to relax knee muscles and makes the legs supple
- encourages blood circulation in the head and is good for wrinkles, a healthy complexion and mental alertness.
- makes the spine supple and pliable
- brings new energy
- relaxes the back and the shoulders
- encourages digestion
- alleviates obesity

II. How to do it

1. Stand with feet together.
2. Slowly lift your hands above the head (Fig. 112).
3. Bend forwards from the hips, keeping the head level. While doing this, first let the head drop forwards and then roll down a vertebra at a time (Fig. 113).
4. Hold your arms next to the ears and for a few seconds let your body hang downwards by its own weight (Fig. 114). Allow the knees to bend if you are uncomfortable.
5. Grasp your ankles or legs, depending on which you can most easily reach. Press your chin into your neck.
6. Bend your elbows outwards, and slowly draw your trunk towards your legs, trying to touch your knees with your forehead (Fig. 115).
7. Stay in this position for a few seconds, breathing gently.
8. Come out of the posture by bending the knees, tucking in the tailbone and slowly rolling back up one vertebra at a time until you are standing upright.
9. Repeat the exercise twice.

III. This is the right way

Do not make any jerky movements in order to bring your forehead closer to your knees.

Be less concerned about how far your hands are from the floor than how far your forehead is away from your knees.

Bending while standing relieves tension in the back and in the hollow of the knees. Simply as a result of the full weight of the whole body hanging downwards, the various parts of the body will be trained and loosened up and eventually you will be able to touch the floor with your hands.

It is important that all movements be carried out slowly.

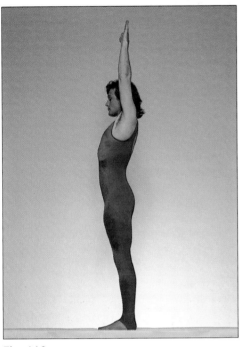

Fig. 112

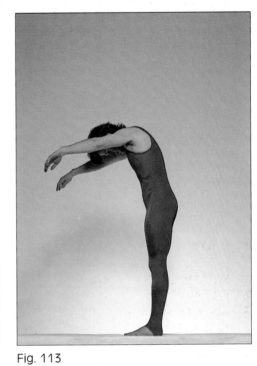

Fig. 113

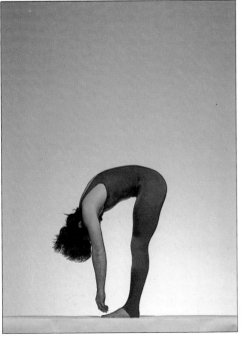

Fig. 114

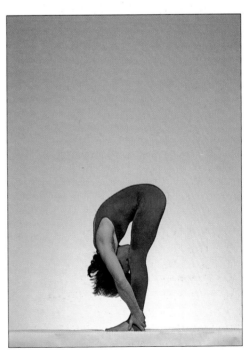

Fig. 115

Corpse (Savasana)

I. What the exercise is good for

The Corpse
- completely relaxes the muscles
- relaxes the whole nervous system
- quietens spirit and soul
- relieves fearful feelings, nervous conditions and sleeplessness
- builds up energy

II. How to do it

1. Lie down on the floor with the legs slightly apart and the arms loose against the body (Fig. 116).
2. Stretch your toes out away from you. Stay like that for 5 seconds and then relax.
3. Bend your toes in the direction of the head by bending the feet at the ankles, remain like this and then relax.
4. Lift your heels a few centimetres from the floor and stretch out your legs, press the hollows of your knees hard against the floor, remain like that and then relax.
5. Stretch out the legs and bring the toes to each other by turning the heels outward, stay like that and then relax.
6. Pull in the buttocks, stay like that and then relax.
7. Pull your stomach inwards and as high as you can, stay like that and then relax.
8. Make your back hollow and stick out the chest, remain so and then relax.
9. Stretch out the arms with the palms downwards, bend the fingers in the direction of the head, remain like that and then relax.
10. Bend the elbows, and bend the hands from the waist outwards in the direction of the shoulders, remain like that and then relax.
11. Form a fist, and spread out the arms slowly with a strong contrary pressure until they are at shoulder height. This strengthens the chest muscles.
12. Pull the shoulder blades together, remain like that and then relax.
13. Pull up the shoulders as high as the ears, remain like that and then relax.
14. Pull the corners of your mouth downwards, remain like that and then relax.
15. Press the tip of the tongue against the gums, remain like that and then relax.
16. Purse your lips, wrinkle your nose, and tightly close your eyes. Remain like that and then relax.
17. Smile with the mouth closed, stretch your face, remain like that and then relax.
18. Yawn, all the time struggling against opening your mouth.
19. Press the back of your head hard against the floor, stay like that and then relax.
20. Furrow the brow, and pull the scalp forwards, remain like that and then relax.
21. Do the eye exercises (page 26).
22. Pull back your head in the direction of the shoulders without moving the rest of the body.
23. Relax. Let yourself sink positively into the floor and lie there for 10 minutes.

III. **This is the right way**

Stay for at least 5 seconds in each final position.
Afterwards relax each time by going back to the original position.
Try to completely relax after this exercise. Put all oppressive thoughts out of your mind – do not weary yourself by 'thinking'. Only let pleasant things file past. Impassively and restfully, watch how they come and go, quite on their own.

The Corpse is a position of total relaxation for the whole body. We hardly ever take real time to relax in this day and age. We read, watch television, sleep, but just lying down does not mean that all the nervous tension that has built up inside us is thereby relieved. Our body must once more learn deep relaxation. After a few weeks of doing this well-balanced exercise you will know how to completely relax without having to go through every procedure in the Corpse.

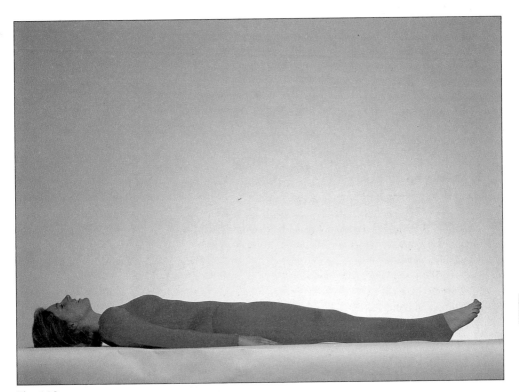

Fig. 116

Sitting Hero (Virasana)

I. What the exercise is good for

The Sitting Hero
- alleviates difficulty with flat feet
- is recommended as a 10-minute exercise when the legs are tired
- lifts the arch of the foot and relaxes it
- reduces pain in the knees and heels
- reduces a feeling of fullness and can be undertaken after eating without danger

II. How to do it

1. Kneel down upright, with the knees together and the feet about half a yard apart (Fig. 117).
2. Lower the body slowly. You can support yourself with the hands (Fig. 118) until you come to sit between the legs.
3. Straighten the back until upright, and let your toes stretch further outwards.

4. Place your hands on the knees with the palms downwards (Fig. 119).
5. Remain in this position for 30 seconds and breathe deeply. The palms face upwards.
6. Stay like this for 30 seconds.
7. Relax.

III. This is the right way

Relax completely in this position. Even after just a short time you can rest. Do not give up if you find it difficult to sit between the feet. Cross over the ankles and sit on them, if it is easier for you. Then try slowly to pull your feet further from each other.
Many people who are constantly on their feet will find this position does them good. In the advanced form, lower yourself back in this sitting position onto the shoulders – to a 'Lying Hero'.

106

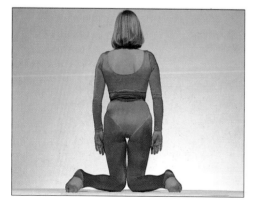

Fig. 117

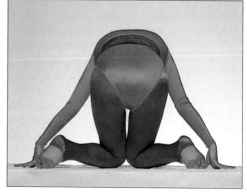

Fig. 118

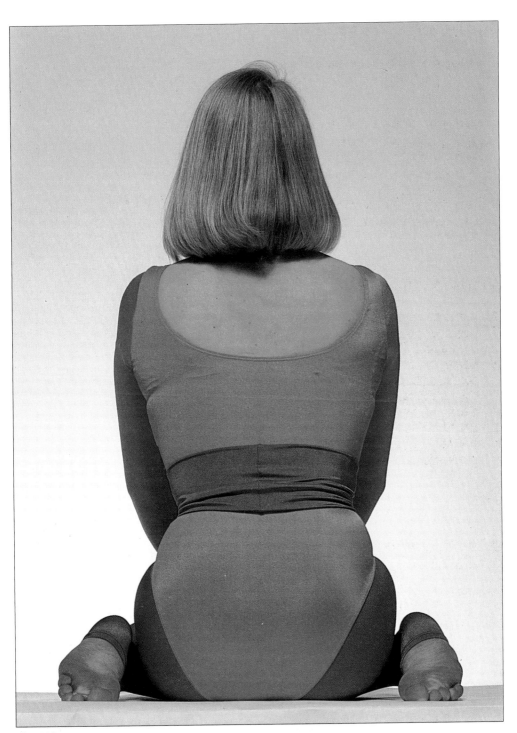

Fig. 119

Scalp massage

I. What the exercise is good for

Scalp massage
- ▶ improves blood circulation of the scalp
- ▶ relaxes
- ▶ makes your hair healthy and shiny
- ▶ helps to prevent hair falling out

II. How to do it

1. Sit comfortably in the Japanese sitting position (see Fig. 56).
2. Grasp your hair completely.
3. Press your fists hard against the scalp, and pull the hair strongly forwards, backwards and to the right and to the left. Undertake this fairly quickly (Fig. 120).
4. Now let your hair go, spread your fingers and place them on the head as though you want to wash the hair (Fig. 121).
5. Press with your fingers quite hard against the scalp and move it all at the same time in different directions (that is better than moving each finger singly).
6. Repeat the exercise several times.

III. This is the right way

Make sure that you hold a thick clump of hair in the hands, otherwise it will hurt. All the time keep your hands quite close to the head.
The massage brings a lovely tingling feeling and removes deep-seated tension.

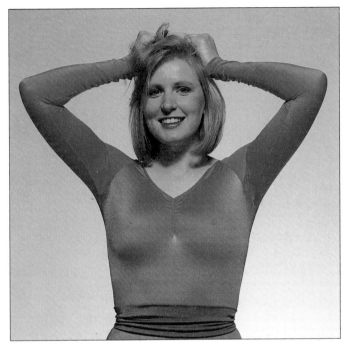

Fig. 120

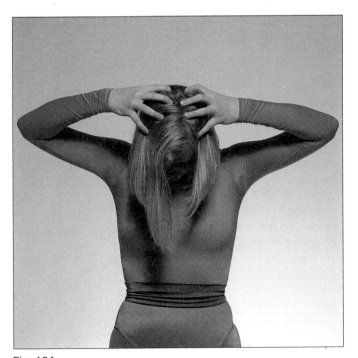

Fig. 121

Twist
(Ardha Matsyendrasana)

I. What the exercise is good for

The Twist
- makes the waist slim
- makes the hip joints supple
- massages the abdominal organs and encourages digestion
- loosens the spine and has a restful effect on the nervous system
- straightens the vertebrae and relaxes
- strengthens the muscles and makes a good figure

II. How to do it

1. Sit yourself on the floor with outstretched legs.
2. Open the legs and place the right foot on the left upper leg. Your right knee must remain firmly on the floor (Fig. 122).
3. Bend the left knee and bring your left foot over your right knee. The knee remains on top (Fig. 123).
4. Place the sole of your left foot completely on the floor. The further back you can move the foot the better.
5. Place your weight now on the pelvis. Support yourself on both hands, so that you do not tip over.
6. Let your left hand support you and place your right arm between the chest and left knee (Fig. 124).
7. Turn your body so that your right shoulder rests on your left knee.
8. Make your right hand into a fist and lead your right arm in a perfectly vertical position over the right knee lying on the floor.
9. Try to grasp the toes of your left foot. As a beginner you will find this quite difficult. If you are not successful, grasp the right knee with your hand (Fig. 125).
10. Now turn the upper part of your body to the left by supporting yourself firmly with your right arm on the left leg.
11. Bend your left arm and place the back of the hand on the outside of the back.
12. Turn your head to the left and look as far as you can to the left (Fig. 126).
13. Remain in this position for 10-30 seconds.
14. Go slowly back into the original position.
15. Repeat the exercise on the other side.

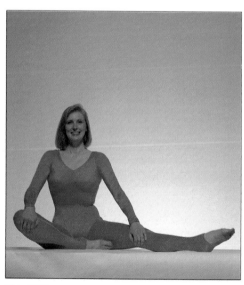

Fig. 122

III. This is the right way

Sit quite forward on your pelvis. Turn yourself with your shoulders and upper leg leaning against the knee. Do not bend your arm in when bringing it over the knee. At the beginning the Twist will appear to be quite difficult. A diagram is easier to follow than many words. When you have found out how it goes, then you will like the Twist. It does you good because it stretches and pulls almost all the muscles in the body. It is even particularly good for the spine.

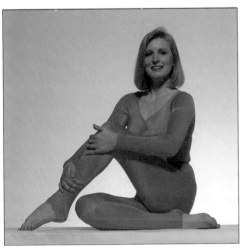

Fig. 123

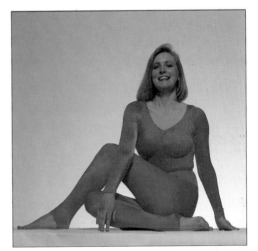

Fig. 124

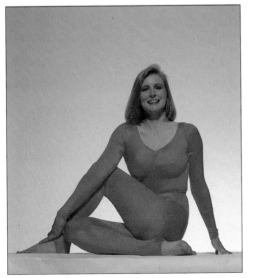

Fig. 125

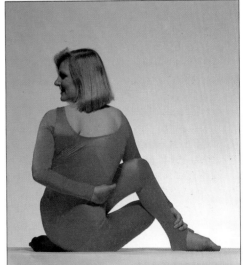

Fig. 126

Toe balance

I. What the exercise is good for

The toe balance
- strengthens the toes
- has a preventative effect on varicose veins
- eases evacuation
- relieves tension
- has a good effect on flat feet
- trains knee joints

II. How to do it (for those who can only stoop on the toes)

1. Squat with the knees wide open. Let your arms hang down between the knees or support them on the knees (Fig. 127).
2. Balance your weight on the toes, afterwards quite slowly on the heels. Go down as low as you can. Try to roll your feet as far as the heels and stay in this position from 5 to 20 seconds.
3. Slowly go back onto the toes. If you need to rest then sit down in between times.
4. Repeat the exercise three times.
5. Always try to close the knees.

III. How to do it (for those who can sit comfortably on their heels)

1. Squat on the floor with the legs wide open. The arms hang down between the knees (Fig. 128).
2. Go slowly onto the tips of your toes and balance for 5-20 seconds.
3. Go back slowly onto your heels.
4. Repeat the exercise three times.
5. Try always to close the knees.

IV. This is the right way

Try out the things that you do not find easy. If you find it easy to balance on your toes, try to move your weight onto your heels and the other way round. Balancing on your toes strengthens not only the toes but the whole foot and the legs. The exercise is very wide in its effectiveness even if it is not immediately discernible.

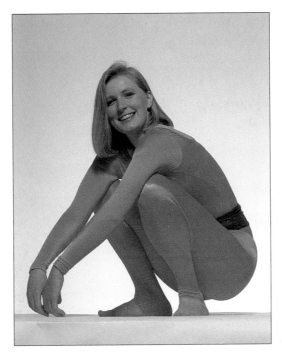

Fig. 127

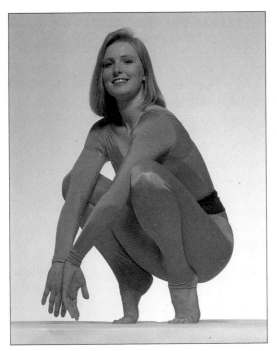

Fig. 128

Toe twist

I. What the exercise is good for

The toe twist
- helps create a slimmer waist
- improves posture
- shapes the legs
- twists the spine like a corkscrew and makes it supple as a result
- strengthens feet and ankles

II. How to do it

1. Sit down in an upright position with the feet close together. The toes should point slightly outwards.
2. Raise yourself slowly on the toes, and stretch the arms out forwards. The thumbs should be hooked together, and the palms should point downwards (Fig. 129).
3. Turn your glance onto the back of your hands, which will ease balance.
4. Bring your arms as much as you can to the side. The movement goes from the waist and the toes remain firmly on the ground.
5. Remain 10–20 seconds in this position, and then turn slowly to the front.
6. Now turn to the other side (Fig. 130). Repeat the exercise twice a day.

III. This is the right way

Do not give up if you lose your balance. Just try again.
Hold your body completely straight, and stick out your chest.
The toe twist has an effect on the whole body. The main benefit can be seen in the posture. Due to the fact that you learn to balance properly, you will be more certain and graceful in your movements.

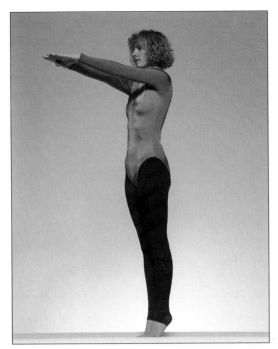

Fig. 129

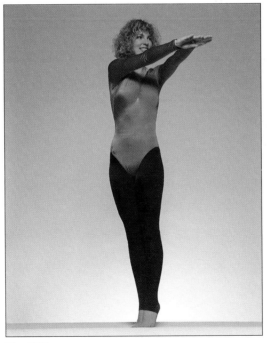

Fig. 130

Rolled-up Leaf (Virasana variation)

I.   What the exercise is good for

The Rolled-up Leaf
- completely relaxes
- creates new energy
- encourages blood circulation in the head and improves the complexion
- relieves tired legs and varicose veins

II.   How to do it

1. Kneel on the ground with your legs closed together.
2. Sit on your heels and place the hands beside them, the tips of the fingers pointing downwards.
3. Bring your head quite slowly onto the ground and leave your hands, palms upward, to move backwards until they rest beside your feet (Fig. 131).
4. Leave your head turned to the side, resting on the floor. Relax completely. Your chest is pressed against the knees.
5. The longer you can remain in this position the better.

III.   This is the right way

Do this exercise whenever you relax or want to replace your energy.
Do not stretch your bottom up too high. Move the whole of the weight onto the legs and heels.
This asana is also called the 'position of the child'. Perhaps it is relaxing simply because it reminds one of being an unborn child in the womb. This exercise has a high therapeutic effect whenever you feel tired or tense.

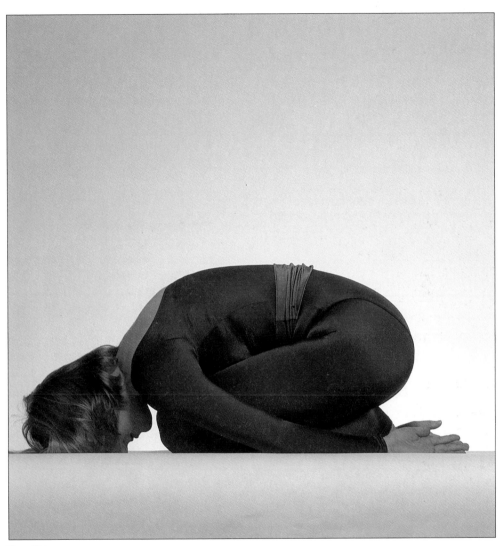

Fig. 131

Breathing Exercises

Alternate nostril breathing (Nadi Sodhana)

I. What the exercise is good for

Alternate nostril breathing
- quietens the nervous system
- helps against sleeplessness
- relaxes and refreshes the body
- purifies the blood and pumps the lungs full of air
- alleviates headaches
- encourages digestion and the appetite
- helps against fear and depression

II. How to do it

1. Sit with a completely straight back in the Japanese sitting position (see Fig. 56).
2. Lift up your right hand and close up the right nostril with the thumb while resting the ring finger against the left nostril.
3. Gently breathe in through the left nostril.
4. Now close both nostrils and hold your breath for about 4 seconds (Fig. 133).
5. Open the right nostril and breathe out slowly through it.
6. Immediately, breathe in through the right nostril.
7. Close both nostrils and hold the breath for up to 4 seconds.
8. Release the left nostril and slowly exhale through it. This provides a complete cycle of breathing.
9. Repeat this cycle five times or for up to 10 minutes, if you suffer from sleeplessness.
10. Breathe in first in a four-four-eight rhythm, later eight-four-eight and, after a few moments, eight-eight-eight.

III. This is the right way

Do not force anything when holding the breath or increasing the rhythm – it must be done slowly and without effort. Breathe rhythmically, slowly and noiselessly.
Always do these breathing exercises when you want to relax and if you are nervous, excited or disturbed.
The meaning of these breathing exercises cannot be emphasised enough. Body and soul stand in a permanent correlation and continually have an influence on each other, more than doctors believed at one time.
The alternate nostril breathing has an incomparably relaxing effect.

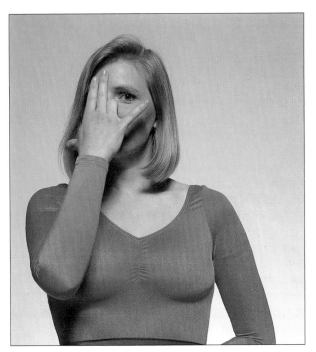

Fig. 132

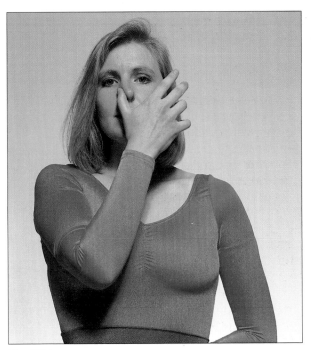

Fig. 133

119

Cleansing breathing (Kapalabhati)

I. What the exercise is good for

Cleansing breathing
- cleans the lungs, sinuses and breathing passages
- alleviates cold
- strengthens the nervous system
- strengthens the lungs, chest and stomach
- purifies the blood and clears the head
- encourages digestion
- encourages the functioning of the liver, spleen and pancreas

II. How to do it

1. Take up the Japanese sitting position with a completely straight back (see Fig. 56), or sit on a chair.
2. Breathe out and then breathe in slowly, relaxing the navel (Fig. 134).
3. Exhale as quickly as you can through both nostrils. This will cause the abdomen to contract (Fig. 135).
4. Relax the abdomen and breathe in gently.
5. Repeat steps 3 and 4 ten times, rhythmically.
6. Stop and take a deep breath before exhaling slowly.
7. Repeat steps 2 to 6 twice.

III. This is the right way

Do not raise the shoulders or try to pull the stomach in. Let the speed of the outward breath do the work and just relax the abdominal wall to allow the in-breath. Once you can do this with ease, a rhythm will develop and you will hear a distinctive 'sawing' sound each time you breathe out. Cleansing breathing is half-way between bellows-breathing, which is fairly difficult to do, and dynamic cleansing breathing. It chases away worries and is a good preparation for tasks demanding energy and care.

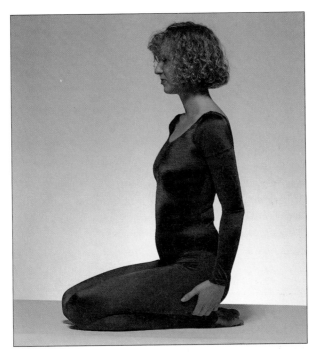

Fig. 134

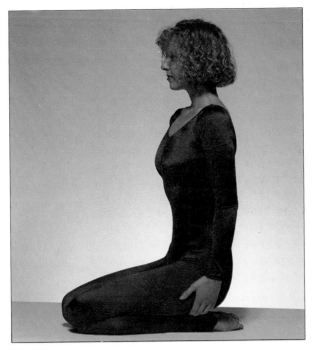

Fig. 135

Full-lung breathing (Ujjayi)

I. What the exercise is good for

Full-lung breathing
▶ brings new energy
▶ purifies the blood
▶ strengthens the chest and the diaphragm
▶ strengthens the lungs and heart
▶ increases resistance to colds
▶ calms the nervous system
▶ encourages digestion
▶ combats lethargy and fatigue
▶ helps against depression

II. How to do it

1. Take up the Japanese sitting position (see Fig. 56), or sit on a chair.
2. Sit upright, then your spine will be straight and you will be able to breathe more easily.
3. Breathe quite slowly, deeply and consciously through the nose.
4. Take 5 seconds to fill the lower parts of the lungs with air by relaxing the navel and allowing the stomach to expand (do not push out) (Fig. 136).
5. Concentrate now for the next 5 seconds on filling the middle ribs to the front, sides and back of the ribcage. Allow the upper part of the chest to pull upwards and sideways into the armpits.
6. Hold your breath for 5 seconds.
7. Breathe out very slowly, drawing in the abdomen, until your lungs are completely empty (Fig. 137).
8. Repeat this exercise four to five times.

III. This is the right way

Find an even rhythm for breathing in and out (this will ensure regularity in breathing).

Do not strain or force the breath and never breathe too deeply – allow a little space at the top of your lungs when you inhale. Keep your tongue and jaw relaxed and your breaths even. Your spine should be upright but relaxed throughout.

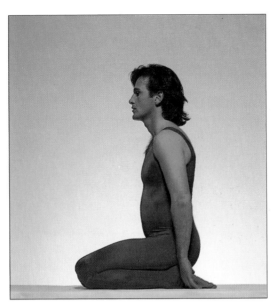

Fig. 136

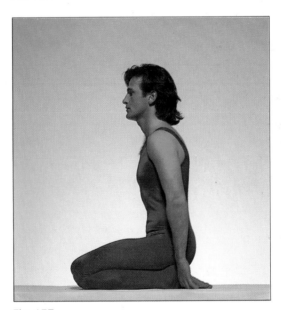

Fig. 137

We need oxygen more than anything else in order to live. Most of us breathe in a flat way, which can be best compared with wolfing down food. Both have a negative effect on health. As a result of deep breathing you will experience a new feeling of vitality! If you consciously breathe correctly, your general state of health can be drastically improved and you will have a completely new outlook on life.

Cooling breathing
(Sitali Pranayama)

I. What the exercise is good for

Cooling breathing
- has a freshening effect and is particularly recommended for high temperatures
- purifies the blood
- helps to prevent breathing difficulties
- encourages digestion
- helps to control the appetite

II. How to do it

1. With a completely straight back take up the Japanese sitting position (see Fig. 56).
2. Stretch out the tongue as far as the lips and make a channel.
3. Breathe, hissing through this channel.
4. Hold your breath for 5 seconds.
5. Breathe out through the nose.
6. Repeat this exercise five times.

III. This is the right way

Practise this breathing exercise if you are healthy – then you will know how to use it when you have a temperature. Do not breathe in too strongly. Take in breath slowly and continuously by extending and retracting the chest and the stomach.

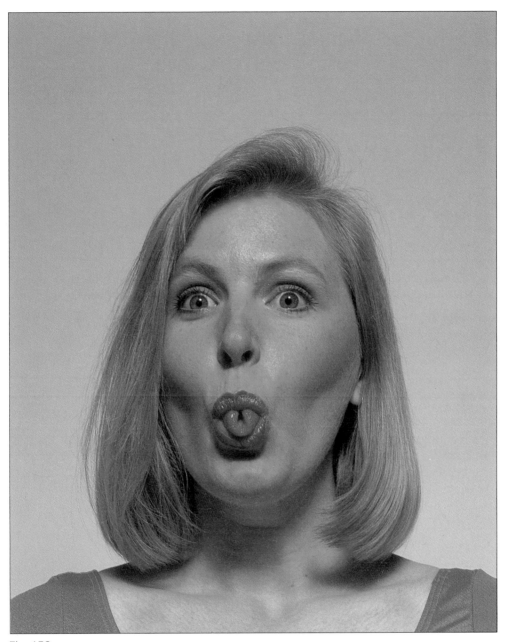

Fig. 138

Exercises for Particular Parts of the Body

These exercises should always be done together with the breathing exercises or in rhythm with breathing. In this way better or more effective results are obtained.

1. Arms and hands

Lifting the arms, Cobra, arm and leg stretching, posture grip, chest expander, Windmill, Bow (advanced), Cat stretching.

2. Eyes

Rolling the eyes, Lion, Candle, headstand, neck rolling.

3. Stomach

Pump (advanced), pulling in the stomach, sitting position, Rock 'n' roll, head to knee stretching, Locust, chest expander, Crossbars, forward-bend sitting, Mountain, crossing the legs.

4. Legs

Toe twist, Sitting Hero, Candle, Tree, arm and leg stretching, Half-lotus, head to knee stretching, forward bending, Bow (advanced), Rolled-up Leaf.

5. Chest and breasts

Chest expander, hands-on-the-wall exercise, posture grip, Cobra, Bow (advanced), Fish, pelvis stretching, Triangle.

6. Heels

Candle, Sitting Hero, Triangle, knee and leg stretching.

7. Feet

Japanese (Diamond) sitting position, Half-lotus, pelvis stretching, Sitting Hero, Toe twist.

8. Bottom

Locust, Cobra, pelvis stretching, Candle, Plough, Pump (advanced), Bow (advanced), head to knee stretching, head-and-trunk raising.

9. Face

Lion, Candle, Plough, forward-bend standing.

10. Hips

Locust, Triangle, Bow (advanced), Warrior, Twist.

11. Knee

Head to knee stretching, knee and leg stretching, Sitting Hero, toe balance, Twist.

12. Ankle

Ankle bends, Triangle, Sitting Hero, Cobra, knee and leg stretching, Crossbars.

13. Neck and chin

Neck roll, chest expander, Fish, Cobra, Plough, Cat stretching.

14. Back and spine

Forward-bend sitting, forward-bend standing, head to knee stretching, Twist, Cat stretching, Plough, Bow (advanced), Cobra, Locust, crossed legs, chest expander, Crossbars, Camel, Pendulum, Pump (advanced).

15. Leg

Knee and leg stretching, spread-leg stretching, head to knee stretching, Triangle, Half-lotus, Sitting Posture, pelvis stretching, arm and leg stretching, Crossbars.

16. Shoulders (posture)

Posture grip, Bell, chest expander, Tree, arm and leg stretching, Bow (advanced), pelvis stretching, Pendulum, Cobra, Plough, arm lifting, Camel.

17. Waist and diaphragm

Twist, Triangle, toe twist, crossed legs, Windmill, pulling in the stomach, Pump.

18. Toes

Toe balance, toe twist, pelvis stretching.

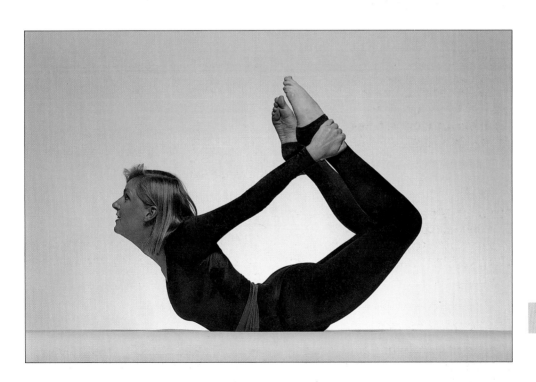

Exercises for Special Problems

1. Anaemia

Candle, forward-bend standing, forward-bend sitting, Corpse, deep breathing.

2. Asthma

Fish, Candle, Mountain, Locust, head to knee stretching, forward-bend sitting, forward-bend standing, Cobra.

3. Back pain

All standing position, Candle, crossed legs, head to knee stretching.

4. Breathing difficulties

Forward-bend sitting, forward-bend standing, Plough, Candle, Mountain, all breathing exercised, Corpse.

5. Circulatory disturbances

Candle, headstand, Pump (advanced), Plough, chest expander, Cobra, Rolled-up Leaf, Pendulum, Mountain, Tree.

6. Colds

Candle, both forward-bends, deep breathing.

7. Constipation

Pulling in the stomach, both forward bends, Twist, Plough, Triangle, Fish, head to knee stretching, Candle, toe balance.

8. Diabetes

Candle, Twist, head to knee stretching, Plough, Fish, Mountain, Locust, forward-bend sitting.

9. Digestion difficulties

Candle, Twist, Cobra, Bow (advanced), Grasshopper, Plough, Mountain, Pump (advanced).

10. Flat feet

Candle, Sitting and Lying Hero, knee and leg stretching.

11. Gall bladder problems

Triangle, both forward bends, Candle, head to knee stretching, Twist, Locust.

12. Haemorrhoids

Fish, Plough, Candle, crossed legs, Grasshopper, Bow (advanced).

13. Headaches

Headstands, Candle, Plough, both forward bends, alternate nostril breathing (without holding the breath), eye rolling, neck rolling.

14. Heart problems

All breathing exercises, especially the deep breathing and alternate nostril breathing (without holding the breath), Corpse.

15. High blood pressure

Plough, head to knee stretching, forward-bend sitting, alternate nostril breathing, Corpse.

16. Intervertebral disc problems

Cat stretching, forward-bend sitting, Locust, all standing positions, Bow (advanced), Camel, Cobra, Fish, Candle.

17. Incontinence

Candle, Sitting and Lying Hero, Fish, knee and leg stretching, pulling in the stomach, Half-lotus.

18. Joint and back pain

Triangle, Mountain, Rolled-up Leaf, Twist, forward-bend standing, Candle, Cobra, Locust.

19. Kidney pain

Candle, all standing positions, Cobra on tip toe, Locust, Bow (advanced), head to knee stretching, forward-bend sitting, knee and leg stretching, spread-leg stretching, crossed legs, Twist, Plough.

20. Lumbago

Plough, Locust, Bow (advanced), Cobra, Corpse.

21. Menstruation problems

Both forward bends, Mountain, Fish, Sitting and Lying Hero, spread-leg stretching, knee and leg stretching, Candle, Cobra, Cat stretching, Triangle.

22. Obesity (weight control)

Plough, Triangle, Cobra, both forward bends, Locust, Twist, Candle.

23. Palpitations

Candle, Plough, both forward bends, Sitting Hero, deep breathing, alternate nostril breathing, Corpse.

24. Prostate difficulties

Crossed legs, forward-bend standing, Locust, Bow (advanced), head to knee stretching, Sitting and Lying Hero, knee and leg stretching.

25. Relaxation

Neck rolling, Lion, Cobra, Candle, Fish, chest expander, Rock 'n' roll, forward-bend sitting, forward-bend standing, knee and leg stretching, head to knee stretching, eye rolling, Rolled-up Leaf, Corpse, deep breathing.

26. Rheumatism

Twist, forward bend, Plough, Mountain, Locust, head to knee stretching, Candle.

27. Rheumatic problems (shoulders)

Bell, Pendulum, chest expander, posture grip.

28. Sciatica

Crossed legs, head to knee stretching, both forward bends, Candle, knee and leg stretching, Locust, Bow (advanced), Cobra, spread-leg stretching.

29. Sexual problems

Candle, pulling in stomach.

30. Sleeplessness

Candle, Cobra, forward-bend sitting, Mountain, Plough, alternate nostril breathing, neck rolling.

31. Tiredness

Candle, headstand, Plough, chest expander, both forward bends, Twist, Rolled-up Leaf, alternate nostril breathing (without holding the breath), deep breathing, ankle bends.

32. Varicose veins

Candle, Sitting and Lying Hero (advanced position), Rolled-up Leaf.

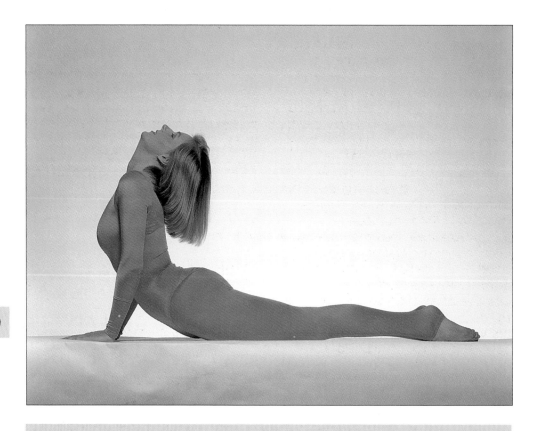

Exercise Programme

A basic programme could look like this:

1. Warm-up – Rock 'n' roll
2. Upside-down position – Candle
3. Gentle loosening up – Lion
4. Bending backwards – Fish
5. Bending forwards – forward-bend sitting
6. Stomach exercise – pulling in the stomach
7. Exercise for legs – arm and leg stretching
8. Turning exercise – Twist
9. Breathing exercise – alternate nostril breathing
10. Relaxation – Rolled-up Leaf

You will certainly have noticed that for every point in the programme a specific exercise is named. You can change these for others, but they should match each of the given points in the programme completely and be in the correct order.
Using the programme scheme reproduced above, it should be possible for you to put together your own programme. Without fail you should take into your daily programme exercised that meet your own particular situation precisely. This could be an exercise for the stomach or to combat headaches, an eye exercise or another exercise you like that is just right for your spirit and body. Should any of the exercises appear to be too difficult for you, then you should try an easier version or another similar one. Always remember, move slowly and do nothing in haste or by force. Stay in the position as long as is comfortable for you.

The most important exercises

1. Rock 'n' roll or chest expander
2. Headstand
3. Candle
4. Pelvis stretching
5. Plough
6. Cobra
7. Forward-bend standing
8. Fish
9. Twist
10. Head to knee stretching
11. Corpse

There are many exercises that are just as important and meaningful as those here named. But for your daily exercise programme, and so that as many organs and muscles as possible are exercised, this combination is the best. How you divide up the time rather depends on how long you take over each exercise.

A 15-minute programme

1. Headstand
2. Candle
3. Cobra
4. Forward-bend sitting
5. Pelvis stretching

If you only have a short time, you should at least do these every day.

You can also replace them with a position you know that does *you* some special good. For example, do the Pump if you want to be rid of the spare tyre around your middle, or pulling in the stomach if you suffer with digestive problems.

Exercise programme to lose weight

1. Warrior
2. Candle
3. Bow (advanced)
4. Plough
5. Fish
6. Pulling in the stomach
7. Pump (advanced)
8. Twist

Add to this list exercises that are particularly aimed at *your trouble spots*. Turn to the chapter on 'Exercises for Particular Parts of the Body', then you will know which exercises to do that are best for you.

Yoga exercises at the office

1. Chest expander
2. Alternate nostril breathing
3. Twist (on a chair)
4. Tree
5. Forward-bend standing
6. Neck rolling
7. Posture grip

Far better than a coffee break is a short energy-providing yoga programme. In some countries the coffee break has been replaced by a half-hour break for exercises, which has led to an astounding increase in production. Try to encourage your colleagues to join you at yoga! You will see how much fun it is.

Yoga for expectant mothers

1. Mountain
2. Deep breathing holding the breath
3. Toe balancing (squatting)
4. Cat stretching (the first two phases)
5. Tree (if necessary using a chair as a support)
6. Knee and leg stretching
7. Hands-on-the-wall exercise

During the first three months of pregnancy you can undertake these exercises with no worry if you have never had a miscarriage. But you should definitely speak to your doctor about it first. The squatting position and the Cat stretching to strengthen the back are especially good for you.

Yoga for children

1. Cat stretching
2. Deep breathing
3. Tree
4. Plough (backwards somersault)
5. Candle
6. Cobra
7. Forward bend
8. Lion
9. Corpse

Children like yoga and are willing and enthusiastic students. As their muscles must always be in motion so that they develop better, one should use a slightly altered version of Hatha yoga. Teach the children when doing the Cat or Lion exercise to behave like a lion or a cat with all the noises that go with them. When doing deep breathing, give them a rubber duck or a rubber boat. It rocks on the stomach as they pull in the stomach and let it out again.

Test the sense of balance of your children by encouraging them to do exercises with their eyes closed. The Plough can be developed further by introducing a backwards somersault. If you lay the children on the floor with the hands at shoulder height and with the fingers at the side of the body, they can push themselves off like that. If by mistake they roll to the side, then they have not pushed hard enough with the hands. With the Corpse exercise they should imagine themselves to be limp rag dolls. Show your children how to do yoga and you will have a lot of fun together.

A divided exercise programme

In the morning
1. Chest expander
2. Deep breathing
3. Forward-bend standing
4. Pelvis stretching
5. Triangle
6. Knee and leg stretching
7. Toe twist
8. Arm and leg stretching
9. Eye rolling

In the evening
1. Pump (advanced)
2. Half-lotus (with forward bend)
3. Candle
4. Lion
5. Twist
6. Pulling in the stomach
7. Bow (advanced)
8. Plough
9. Cobra

10. Neck rolling
11. Alternate nostril breathing
12. Corpse

Yoga for those who want to give up smoking

The best method of kicking the smoking habit is to accustom your body to correct breathing. Do the following breathing exercises in the fresh air:
1. Dynamic cleansing breathing
2. Deep breathing
3. Alternate nostril breathing
4. Cooling breathing

The first of these two exercises you should do both at the beginning and at the end of your exercise programme. Do these exercises every time you are in the fresh air and every time you really want to smoke. Just before going to sleep you should do the alternate nostril breathing exercise. If you have been a strong smoker over many years, at the beginning you may get slightly dizzy. This is due to an excess of oxygen but is no cause for worry. The dizziness will disappear the more your body turns to breathing habits that are healthy and will lengthen your life.

Release Yoga

Just as yoga has nothing to do with yoghurt or Yo-Yos, so here release yoga has nothing to do with the release mechanism of a camera or the trigger of a pistol. Instead, this expression means that the environmental stimulation of everyday life should trigger off the thought: 'Ah, this is the right time to do…[a well loved yoga exercise].' For example, when driving the car or sitting as a passenger and you come to a red light you will be reminded that now is the time to do an exercise for the chest, something against crease marks or a sore throat. In other words, press your hands against the steering wheel, or do the Lion exercise! By doing this exercise you can drive through the city traffic without being affected by the aggression it can cause.

Do you see the tremendous possibilities? You can do your yoga exercises without a lot of effort *any time* and *anywhere*! I am often asked how many hours I do yoga. My answer is: 24 hours, at any time of the day or night!

I am certain that in practising release yoga you will discover your own exercises that are not on my lists.

1. *On waking*
Stretching exercise: Stretch sideways in bed with your shoulders held straight. Try to stretch out both hands alternately, as though you were about to grasp your feet.

2. *When brushing your teeth*
Alternate leg stretching: Place one foot on the lid of the toilet, the window sill or the wash-basin, bend the leg on which you are standing up and down, and clean your teeth at the same time. Change the legs over.

3. *When brushing your hair*
Forwards bend: When doing this bend keep the knees straight and brush your hair, the wrists being loose. Try with each brush movement to bend further forwards.

4. *In the kitchen*
Squatting: Squat for example when you need to peel something. Stand on your toes if you need to reach for something in a cupboard. Stand with your back to the cupboard and go slowly on to the tips of your toes, at the same time turning the upper part of your body towards the cupboard.

5. *While eating*
Muscle exercises: Get your partner to sit opposite you. Pull off your shoes and place your feet in the lap of your partner. Or tighten and relax the muscles of your bottom. Repeat this several times.

6. *At the desk*

Chest expander sitting: Sit on the edge of the chair with legs apart. The hands are folded behind the back. Bend forwards breathing out at the same time and stretch your hands as far as possible upwards.

7. *When telephoning*

Balancing: Stand in the Tree position on one leg and bring the other leg with the foot to the inside of the thigh. Hold this position for as long as you can. If necessary you can balance yourself by gently leaning on a wall.

8. *When lifting a heavy object*

Drawing in the stomach: Bend forwards. At the same time, breathe out, relax and let the stomach draw itself in. Hold this position for a second, then breathe in again and relax while letting the stomach expand. This exercise works wonders with the muscles and the digestion.

9. *In front of the television*

Sitting: Sit so that your knees are bent only as much as having the feet flat on the ground will allow. Cross over the arms behind the head, then place them back again. When doing this exercise beginners can hook their feet under a piece of furniture and rest on one elbow.

Bow position (Seesaw): Lie on your stomach on the floor and grasp the ankles with the hands or with the help of loops breathe out and press your ankles away from the hands while all the time keeping the head upright. Breathe deeply all the time so that the body, as a result of the breathing movement, bobs up and down. Relax and repeat the exercise.

Spread-leg stretching while sitting: Spread the legs as wide apart as possible. Then bend the body forwards with the wrists placed together and the elbows bent, place the hands on the floor and place the head in the cupped hands. Hold this position as long as possible.

Crossed legs: Lie down on the floor in such a way that the crossed legs can be hooked somewhere as you face the television. Hold this position as long as you can.

10. *While waiting at traffic lights*

Hands-on-the-wall (steering wheel): Bend the elbows slowly and press against the forward movement of the body until the head touches the steering wheel. Then return slowly to the position from which you began.

11. *In a car, bus or aeroplane*

Relaxation exercises: Press your head against the back-rest and hold this position for a short time. Place your hands on the knees as though about to get up. Tense and then relax the various groups of muscles. Move our shoulders upwards, backwards, forwards, and in a circle. Let your head go round in a circle.

Yoga Exercises for People Over 50

Many of the health problems that increase as one gets older can be avoided through yoga exercises and proper diet. Go through the following list and choose the exercises that suit you best. In any case, speak first with your doctor.

Breathing difficulties: Breathing problems are often a result of bad posture (which gets worse with age). They also frequently arise through smoking, which is bad not only for the lungs but also the throat, mouth and nose. Give up smoking and then do the Half-lotus with deep breathing.

Eye problems: Although these problems cannot be avoided altogether as a result of yoga exercises and taking vitamins A and B_2, the effect can be minimised. A lack of vitamin A leads to sensitivity to light, night blindness, tiredness of the eyes, unclear vision and burning of the eyes.

Haemorrhoids: Haemorrhoids can be very painful, so constipation should be avoided at all costs. The consumption of solids should be kept to a minimum, while on the other hand the consumption of fluids should be increased. To ease the stool you should have a low footstool in the bathroom on which to place one foot while sitting back as far as possible. After a successful stool the haemorrhoids hanging out should be pushed back and then the buttocks clenched together several times. To alleviate the pain, I suggest above all the Fish and the Candle.

Heart disease: Heart disease imposes severe restrictions on the health in middle and old age. Although there are many causes of heart disease some of them can be avoided altogether. Heart specialists advise cutting out three of the main risk factors as soon as there are danger signs, and before this leads to hardening of the arteries. The first factor is a high cholesterol level, the second high blood pressure and the third is smoking. Although it is not yet clear what effect smoking has, it is known that it increases the amount of carbonmonoxide in the blood, and that it separates important oxygen from the haemoglobin (colouring agent of the red blood corpuscles) and so reduces the supply of oxygen to the body cells and blood vessels. In addition, many believe that smoking weakens the heart muscles. There are a number of other secondary risk factors such as diabetes, overweight, strong alcohol consumption, lack of exercise, stress and exhaustion. Most of these factors can be eliminated by changing one's life-style and through proper exercise. Add to your yoga exercises additional exercise such as walking or swimming to strengthen your heart. Keep the blood pressure low by breathing exercises and meditation. If you suffer with heart problems you should avoid upside down yoga exercises unless specifically recommended by a doctor. To avoid heart disease you should practise deep breathing and alternate nostril breathing without holding the breath, and the Corpse.

High blood pressure: High blood pressure is a high risk factor for those with heart disease and can be caused by tension, excitement and stress. In addition, there are many physical reasons such as a high intake of salt and overweight.

Doctors recommend patients with high blood pressure to eat a salt-free diet, have physical exercise and plenty of rest, and to give up smoking. If you suffer with high blood pressure you should have your blood pressure measured regularly. Food scientists have discovered that people with high blood pressure experience an easing of their condition after a diet high in protein, vitamin B and lecithin. Smoking is not only connected with lung cancer, breathing problems and mouth cancer but it is also one of the three high risk factors for heart and vascular disease. The following exercises help against high blood pressure: forward-bend sitting, alternate nostril breathing and the Corpse.

High blood pressure, heart attack, gallstones, gout, diabetes and the effects of ageing: All these problems are made worse by physical inactivity and overweight. The resulting pain can sometimes be alleviated or can even be totally eliminated, by exercise and losing weight. The Fish and the Plough exercises help you to lose weight as they stimulate the thyroid gland.

Sciatica: Sciatica makes itself felt by pain from the large leg nerve. Such a pain can sometimes be caused by straining a pelvis joint or problems with a disc. With the onset of sciatica you should visit a chiropractor or osteopath. Also take vitamins of the B group and do such exercises as knee and leg stretching and forward bends. Rest a lot.

Brittle bones (osteoporosis): Many doctors feel that weight-bearing exercise is good for bones and joints and many yoga postures and sequences can build bone density. However, anyone with osteoporosis should consult a doctor before beginning yoga.

Varicose veins: Varicose veins can be hereditary or caused by excess weight, tight clothing and crossing the legs when sitting. The condition can be alleviated to some extent by wearing looser clothing, taking vitamins B, C and D, doing suitable exercises, putting the feet up when sitting and controlling the weight. A good exercise to combat varicose veins is to stand on tiptoe on each step when going upstairs. In addition, you can do a series of squat positions or other exercises that will strengthen calf muscles. Especially helpful are the upside-down yoga exercises.

Low blood sugar (hypoglycaemia): This disease leads to a large appetite, tiredness and exhaustion, headaches, dizziness, nervousness, fearful feelings and even unconsciousness. Whereas a low blood sugar condition can be caused by hormonal or mental imbalance, it is usually due to an excessive intake of carbohydrates (starch and sugar) and a lack of panthothenic acid. What can be helpful here is a diet high in protein, low in carbohydrates and rich in vitamins of the B complex and potassium. Avoid sugar and foods with a high sugar content. In addition, vitamin C is a great help in acute attacks – it strengthens exhausted suprarenal glands.

Prostate infections: Difficulties here can be alleviated by a balanced diet including a high content of vitamin A, vitamins of the B complex and vitamin C. To ensure a healthy prostate, unsaturated fatty acids (vegetable oils) are important. Many doctors forbid alcohol and very spicy foods in prostate cases. The knee and leg stretching is a good exercise here.

Back pains: Back pain can be brought on by bad posture, inactivity, lifting and carrying heavy objects in an awkward way and overweight. To alleviate or prevent back pain, you should do exercises like the Cobra, pulling in the stomach, pelvis stretching and the Pendulum.

Sleeplessness: Disturbed sleep can often be traced back to bad diet, too much caffeine intake (the one cup of coffee in the afternoon is often the villain), stress, lack of physical exercise and mental problems. Often it is a vicious circle that is difficult to break because of fear of not being able to sleep. Try a cup of camomile tea or hot milk, a short walk, a warm foot-bath or a good book. The chest expander, headstand or Candle, neck rolling, Fish, Plough, Twist, alternate nostril breathing and the Corpse are relaxing exercises to put you to sleep.

Stroke: Blood analysis of stroke patients has revealed that of this group 80 per cent suffer from a lack of vitamin E. We recommend a programme of yoga exercises, avoiding, however, all upside-down exercises without previously speaking to your doctor.

Constipation: Constipation can be avoided by a good diet containing sufficient protein and roughage. In addition, natural foods that help with this problem are, for example, fresh fruit and wholegrain cereals. It is important to get physical exercise. Exercise with the forward bends, the Twist, the Plough, the Fish, the Candle and pulling in the stomach. Walk regularly.

Dropsy (oedema): Dropsy can be caused by water that, due to lack of potassium is retained in the cells. Often an ill-balanced diet, high sugar and sale consumption and the intake of diuretic agents can lead to dropsy. The signs are swollen eyes and thick ankles. Medicines to take away the excess water artificially are not a healthy long-term solution, but only make things worse by removing potassium from the body. It is preferable to use more natural means of achieving a diuretic effect, such as potassium chloride, vegetable oil, protein, vitamin B, unsalted peanuts, melons, bananas, figs, plums, olives, almonds or potatoes. As exercises for anyone with dropsy I recommend the Candle, crossed legs, Twist, Plough, Locust, knee and leg stretching, forward bends and the Cobra.

Menopause problems: To quieten the nerves it is sometimes advisable for the body to take in supplementary doses of calcium, magnesium or phosphorus. In addition, your diet should contain plenty of calcium, in order to support the fluid balance in the body. Overweight, which is often a result of depression, can be reduced by suitable exercises. A well-balanced diet with lots of B complex vitamins can help women over this difficult time. If you are taking feminine hormones you should increase your intake of vitamin E. Although the menopause in men does not have such a strong physical effect, it can affect the psyche. As in women, there is a fundamental change in the production of sex hormones. Often during this time men feel themselves to be less 'manly' and can at times seek to prove their manliness through excessive sexual activity, which can then lead to impotence.

For both sexes the following programme is equally recommended: Cat stretching, the Candle, the Cobra, forward-bend sitting, Twist, pelvis stretching, deep breathing, the Corpse.

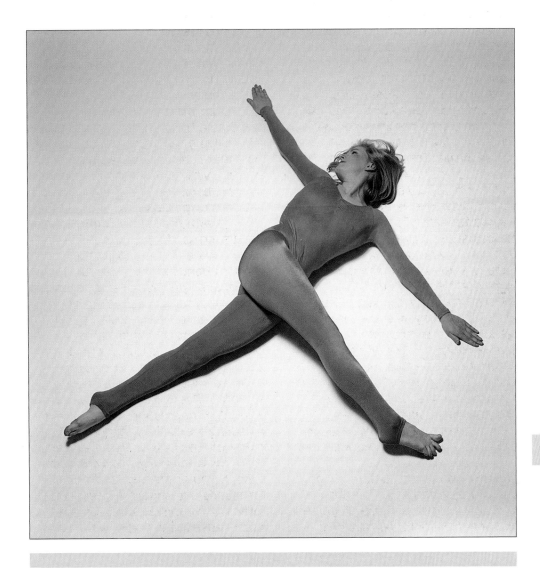

In the Case of Back Problems Prevention is Better than Cure

If you have a weak back, you should strengthen it through exercises. In the case of back pain, you should ask the doctor what exercises are suitable for you. If you want to know how to keep your back healthy, practise yoga and keep to the following advice:

1. Try to avoid standing for long periods of time as this puts pressure on the lumbar vertebrae.
2. If you are compelled to stand for a long time, place your foot on a stool and rest your elbow on the bent knee. This will keep the back straight.
3. Sleep on a firm mattress. Try not to sleep on your stomach. If you sleep on your back, as well as having a pillow for your head push one under your knees. However, it is best if you sleep on your side with bent knees.
4. When you wake in the morning, roll over on the side, swing your legs from the bed and then lift yourself to a sitting position using your arms. This way of getting up minimises the pressure on the spine.
5. If you are lying or sitting in bed watching the television, do not hold your head at a sharp angle.
6. To lift up heavy objects, bend at the knees in order to avoid straining the muscles, discs and tendons.
7. Cross your legs at the ankles only. Crossing the legs at the knees will increase the problems for back-

pain sufferers and hinder the circulation of the blood to the legs, which can lead to varicose veins, circulatory problems and swollen ankles.

8. Always sit in firmly upholstered armchairs with a straight back. Avoid soft armchairs and sofas.
9. Force nothing. Get to know your physical limits and build up your strength only gradually.
10. If necessary, try to lose weight. Overweight places a burden on the spine, legs and heart.
11. Always keep yourself physically active. If you have to do something sitting down, always stand up for a break and walk about. Try to slip in a short walk or a yoga exercise first thing in the morning or in the evening – even if it is only for 10 minutes.
12. Always tip your body forwards when walking and standing. In this way the spine is kept upright, the bottom and stomach muscles are strengthened and, besides this, pain in the lower spinal region is reduced. This way of walking is the best and certainly the most attractive.
13. If you have to lift or carry something or straighten your legs, you should always tense the stomach and bottom muscles, press the pelvis forwards and at the same time breathe out.
14. Finish an exercise just as slowly as you began it.

15. Provided you have no varicose veins, you should go into a squat as often as you can in order to strengthen the leg muscles.
16. Place one foot on a low stool if you have to bend from the waist forwards (when washing dishes or brushing teeth).
17. Never straighten the knee completely, but hold it just slightly bent.
18. Always keep yourself warm to prevent tense and hardened muscles. Take warm baths and wear warm clothing. Use a hot water-bottle or heated cushion.
19. Your next present should be a rocking chair – even if you have to buy it yourself. As a result of the gentle rocking movement, the circulation of the blood is improved and the spine kept supple. The best rocking chairs have a foot support.
20. Buy a low footstool for your bathroom. You will discover that bowel movements are made easier if you place one foot on a stool.
21. Only wear shoes with flat heels, thick soles and plenty of room for the toes. High heels lead to painful tension and bad posture.
22. Do not ignore pain signals. Stay in the sleeping position, stretch yourself slowly, put on something warm and consult a doctor or chiropractor.
23. If you suffer with back pain then you should only drive if you can lean on a back-rest. Avoid long flights. Do not sit in chairs that have a very straight back. When sitting, slip a cushion behind your back.

24. In order to support your body when sneezing, laughing or coughing you should straighten your hands and press them against your stomach.
25. Never support anything with your hips. Do not lean things against your hips. The shoulders are much better suited to carrying things than the hips. Always remember that the pelvis should be pressed forward, in order to keep the spine straight. Ideally you should always stand with slightly bent knees, the feet slightly apart and the chest held high. Breathe deeply, hold the chin and head high and the shoulders down. Tense the stomach muscles and pull the buttocks together.
26. Just for women. Back pain can have a gynaecological cause. Ask your doctor. Tampons sometimes cause back pain. in this case it is better if you use sanitary towels.

Exercise plans

If you do not keep your back in training it can easily become stiff and painful. When not used, muscles shrink and lose their elasticity, so they lose their agility. In order to remain agile, it is very important to use these muscles and to stretch them. Always consult a doctor or chiropractor as to which exercises best suit you.

Exercises to loosen stiff muscles

Alternate leg stretching
Crossbars
Camel
Spread-leg stretching
Cobra
Candle
Head to knee stretching
Crossed legs

Against arthritis of the spine

Bell
Pendulum

In the case of pain in the hips

Candle
Knee and leg stretching
Spread-leg stretching

Relief of severe back pain

Pelvis stretching
Head to knee stretching

In the case of back injuries and posture damage

Bell
Bow (advanced)
Camel
Crossed legs

Exercises for strengthening the back muscles

Pendulum
Head-and-trunk raising
Spread-leg stretching

Exercises for keeping the back healthy

Rock 'n' roll
Crossbars
Pelvis stretching
Head to knee stretching
Cobra

Exercises for relieving tension

Bow (advanced)
Twist
Alternate leg stretching
Deep forward bends

Exercises the intervertebral discs

Locust
Bow (advanced)
Cobra

Keeping a straight back

Cobra
Twist

foulsham

The Publishing House
Bennetts Close, Cippenham, Slough, Berks SL1 5AP

ISBN 0–572–02802–4

First published as *Yoga for Everyone*
Originally published by Falken-Verlag GmbH,
Niedernhausen TS, Germany.
Photographs copyright © Falken-Verlag.

The exercises in this book are safe provided the
instructions are followed carefully. The authors
and publishers are followed carefully. The authors
and publishers disclaim all liability arising from the
use of the information. If you have any doubts
about the suitability of any of the exercises,
consult a doctor.

Printed in Great Britain
by Bath Press, Glasgow